'Kudos to the editors and all the authors of this timely and i intersectionality and group analysis. Each chapter examines their experiences of the constraints and restraints of the tripartite matrix in their training and colleagueship within the profession. Readers are asked to consider how their own identities and internalized privileges inform how they conduct their groups. A bold and courageous invitation!'

Richard Beck, *LCSW, BCD, CGP, AGPA-F; Immediate Past President, IAGP; Senior Lecturer, Columbia University School of Social Work; Honorary Member, Italian Society for Psychosomatic Medicine; Lecturer in Social Work in Psychiatry (Voluntary) Weill Cornell Medicine*

'This exciting and innovative volume highlights the vitality of new currents in group analytic thinking and practice that speaks to urgent sociopolitical agendas for change. Compelling and thought-provoking, its eight innovative, scholarly, but above all practice-focused chapters invite and inspire engagement and activism that both consolidate the core contributions of group analysis and also transform it. This will be a core text for all trainees in psychotherapy and counselling.'

Professor Erica Burman, *Professor of Education, Manchester Institute of Education, UK*

'*Intersectionality and Group Analysis* is an inspiring, creative, and innovative paradigm change to decolonize group analytic theory and practice and to allow for group polyphonic spaces. It promises to enable anti-racist therapeutic practice in clinics and in training. A highly relevant and much-needed impulse for the advancement of group analysis in a globalized world.'

Dr Elisabeth Rohr, *Professor, Intercultural Education, Philipps-University Marburg, Germany (until 2013); group analytical trainer, consultant and supervisor in national and international fields of work*

'The authors together flesh out intersectionality as a necessarily embodied and collective approach to interpreting and changing the world, making the book an invaluable conceptual resource and call to action for group analysts, for every analyst.'

Professor Ian Parker, *Secretary, Manchester Psychoanalytic Matrix, UK*

'Finally! Group analysis, in theory and practice, is making space for people with historically marginalized identities. This important network of authors has unapologetically and beautifully captured the simultaneously painful and generative experience of being the Other, not just subjectively but also structurally. They argue that until the many forms of structural oppression are accounted for and centred in our work, psychoanalysis and psychotherapy will continue to be for a select privileged group. Understanding intersectionality is at the heart of offering ethical, humane, compassionate, and skilful care for everyone.'

Kavita Avula, *Psy.D.; President, Therapists Beyond Borders; Soundview School Board of Trustees; Vice President, National Group Psychotherapy Institute; Past President, Dean Puget Sound Group Psychotherapy Network*

Intersectionality and Group Analysis

Drawing on clinical practice, this book explores how the Black feminist idea of intersectionality is vital to all group work practices, including group analysis.

Intersectionality enables the exploration of power, position, and privilege in group work; this volume is an argument for the 'decolonizing' of therapeutic group training, practice, and institutional traditions. The wide range of contributors discuss the impact of intersectionality on their work within group analysis, from clinical examples to theoretical reflections. Chapters span topics such as leadership, racism, working with survivors of sexual violence, and the experience of being a political refugee. *Intersectionality and Group Analysis* provides a space to develop clinically relevant theory for the future and includes an accessible introduction to the concepts of intersectionality.

This essential text will be key reading for group analysts, other professionals working with and within groups, and readers looking to learn more about enhancing diversity within structures and organizations.

Suryia Nayak, PhD is Senior Lecturer in Social Work at the University of Salford, UK. She is a group analyst and feminist activist and has over 40 years of experience applying intersectionality in her work to end violence against women and girls, the trauma of forced migration, and the impact of colonization.

Alasdair Forrest, MRCPsych is a Group Analyst. He is Consultant Forensic Psychiatrist and Medical Psychotherapist at the Royal Cornhill Hospital, Scotland, UK. He chairs the Faculty of Medical Psychotherapy of the Royal College of Psychiatrists in Scotland and the training committee of the Glasgow Foundation Course in Group Analysis.

The New International Library of Group Analysis (NILGA)
Series Editor: Earl Hopper

Drawing on the seminal ideas of British, European and American group analysts, psychoanalysts, social psychologists and social scientists, the books in this series focus on the study of small and large groups, organisations and other social systems, and on the study of the transpersonal and transgenerational sociality of human nature. NILGA books will be required reading for the members of professional organisations in the field of group analysis, psychoanalysis, and related social sciences. They will be indispensable for the "formation" of students of psychotherapy, whether they are mainly interested in clinical work with patients or in consultancy to teams and organisational clients within the private and public sectors.

Recent titles in the series include:

A Psychotherapist Paints
Insights from the Border of Art and Psychotherapy
Morris Nitsun

Group Analysis throughout the Life Cycle
Foulkes Revisited from a Group Attachment and Developmental Perspective
Arturo Ezquerro and Maria Cañete

The Tripartite Matrix in the Developing Theory and Expanding Practice of Group Analysis
The Social Unconscious in Persons, Groups and Societies: Volume 4
Edited by Earl Hopper

Intersectionality and Group Analysis
Explorations of Power, Privilege, and Position in Group Therapy
Edited by Suryia Nayak and Alasdair Forrest

For more information about this series, please visit: www.routledge.com/Routledge-Handbooks-in-Religion/book-series

Intersectionality and Group Analysis

Explorations of Power, Privilege, and Position in Group Therapy

Edited by Suryia Nayak and
Alasdair Forrest

Routledge
Taylor & Francis Group
LONDON AND NEW YORK

Designed cover image: *Pandora's Box*, image by Claire Bacha, September 2021, digital photograph.

First published 2024
by Routledge
4 Park Square, Milton Park, Abingdon, Oxon OX14 4RN

and by Routledge
605 Third Avenue, New York, NY 10158

Routledge is an imprint of the Taylor & Francis Group, an informa business

British Library Cataloguing-in-Publication Data
A catalogue record for this book is available from the British Library

ISBN: 978-1-032-14071-1 (hbk)
ISBN: 978-1-032-14073-5 (pbk)
ISBN: 978-1-003-23221-6 (ebk)

DOI: 10.4324/9781003232216

Typeset in Times New Roman
by Apex CoVantage, LLC

In memory of Claire Bacha

Contents

Contributors

Anne Aiyegbusi is a group analyst, forensic psychotherapist, and registered mental health nurse. She works part-time as a principal psychotherapist and group analyst at Oxford NHS Foundation Trust. She is also a Director of Psychological Approaches CIC, an independent training and consultancy company. She is a member of the Board of Trustees for the Institute of Group Analysis, where she is the member for anti-discrimination and intersectionality.

Daniel Anderson is a consultant psychiatrist, group analyst, and psychodynamic psychotherapist working in the NHS at The Christie NHS Foundation Trust, Manchester, in the Department of Psycho-oncology, and in private practice. Dan is also an honorary clinical reader (associate professor) in psychotherapy at the University of Central Lancashire, England. Dan completed his PhD at the University of Manchester's Institute of Education and consequently authored the book *The Body of the Group: Sexuality and Gender in Group Analysis*. He is the chair of the charity and psychotherapy training organization Group Analysis North.

Claire Bacha was a psychotherapist and group analyst in private practice in Manchester. She was one of the founder students of the Manchester Qualifying Course and worked on the Manchester Courses from 1996 to 2021 in various capacities. Claire was active in the Power, Position, and Privilege movement at the Institute of Group Analysis. Claire's book *The Group Dimension*, which summarises her lifetime's thinking, is to be published posthumously. In downtime, she played with abstract photography.

Anthea Benjamin is a UKCP/BACP registered Integrative Arts Psychotherapist, Adolescent Psychotherapist, Group Analyst, Supervisor, trainer, and organizational consultant. Anthea has worked extensively with children, adolescents, adults, families, couples, and groups for over 20 years in various settings, including schools, community projects, and within the NHS. Anthea also offers therapeutic services such as self-reflective groups and team supervision both in organizations and within her private practice in south London. Anthea has a special interest in racial trauma, particularly working with racial trauma in the body.

Dick Blackwell is a Group Analyst, Family Therapist, and Organisation Consultant; Associate Editor of *Group Analysis*; a graduate of Business Management, he studied Physical Education, then worked as a researcher on the youth and community work project Black Youth in the Inner City before training in group analysis and family therapy. He has been coordinator of volunteer counsellors and psychotherapists at the Medical Foundation for the Care of Victims of Torture, Consultant Group and Family Therapist to Baobab Centre for Young Survivors in Exile, and Founder and Director of the Centre for Psychotherapy and Human Rights; author of *Counselling and Psychotherapy with Refugees*; co-author of *Far from the Battle but Still at War: Troubled Refugee Children in Schools*; and has written extensively on psychotherapy, culture, and politics. In the early 1970s, he was a 'student power' activist and later a contributor to the 'Occupy' movement. He now consults for a community project generated by the Grenfell community in the aftermath of the fire, is a founding member of the 'Decolonising Group Analysis Group', and a seminar conductor on the IGA (UK)s London qualifying course.

Farideh Dizadji is a political refugee in exile since 1984, an intersectional internationalist, feminist, and socialist, which constitutes her group analytic positionality. Farideh is a group analyst, psychotherapist, clinical supervisor, and organizational consultant. Farideh is a qualified member of the Institute of Group Analysis and a member of the Group Analytical Society International. Farideh has worked with the Medical Foundation for the Care of Victims of Torture and was the clinical director of Nafsiyat, a clinical supervisor at the Women's Therapy Centre, and the clinical director of Kids Company's principal London centre. Farideh holds a private practice.

Reem Shelhi is a neurodiverse Anglo-Arab queer Contemporary Psychotherapist, Group Analyst, and Clinical Supervisor with a unique intersectional history providing a rich foundation for her work on identity, sexuality, oppression, and existential issues around loss, grief, and the search for meaning. Her current project, www.alloneworld.org, is a politically inflected enterprise exploring the paradoxical relationship between the individual and society, looking at ways which could potentially yield innovative approaches to working with group analysis in an increasingly complex and fragmented world. Her specific work with queer Arab Muslims underscores a commitment to providing culturally sensitive and inclusive care, recognizing the unique challenges faced by this particular community.

Preface

I am privileged to have been able to use the influence – if not the power – afforded by my position as Editor of the New International Library of Group Analysis to facilitate the publication by Routledge of this virtually unique volume of passionate essays in the application of group analytic theory to the study of intersectionality not only in the foundation matrix of our contextual society but also in the dynamic matrices of our two intertwined professional organizations, i.e., the Institute of Group Analysis (UK) and the Group Analytic Society International, as well as of many other organizations in the mental health field in England and in other countries. Deeply concerned with the grotesque distortions of psychic life inherent in the hierarchies of various kinds of power, the authors of these chapters discuss in personal and academically informed ways the insults perpetrated by the inequalities and inequities associated with many socially unconscious facts, factors, and processes.

It is painfully ironic that in phases of rebellious change, those societies and organizations that have instigated and nourished change are also those whose younger members are most aggrieved by the failures of their "parents" to realise their aims and expectations. Nonetheless, those who were at the vanguard must take responsibility for their failures, as will, in due course, their "children".

In this context, I (e.g., Hopper, 2023a) have often defined 'mature hope' as the ability and willingness to exercise the transcendent imagination. I have also argued that this depends on authentic dialogue across the generations and across the boundaries that define self and others, for example, those of stratification, race, ethnicity, sex, and gender. However, we must not neglect the vicissitudes of personal matrices and the personification of social facts, factors, and processes (Hopper, 2023b). Activism is always Janus-faced towards both the internal and external worlds. We are tasked with the challenge to make creative use of traumatogenic processes that are rooted in failed dependency on our elders who have delivered less than what they promised.

Dr Suryia Nayak and Dr Alasdair Forrest are to be congratulated for gathering and holding together a network of colleagues who share their hopes for Group Analysis. They encourage us to improve, develop, and extend our clinical and political projects. Although further work and study are necessary, we must strive not to fail them, but when we do, to fail them better.

References

Hopper, E. (2023a). A Hopeful Memoir of the 'Baldwin/Buckley' Debate in 1965, in Cambridge, England. *Forum: Journal of International Association for Group Psychotherapy and Group Processes*, July, 52–57. https://iagp.com/wp-content/uploads/2023/07/FORUM_11_FINAL.pdf

Hopper, E. (ed.) (2023b) *The Tripartite Matrix in the Developing Theory and Expanding Practice of Group Analysis: The Social Unconscious in Persons, Groups and Societies: Volume 4*. London: Routledge.

Introduction

Putting Intersectionality to Work

Suryia Nayak

Intersectionality is necessary for therapeutic work. Whilst this book focusses on group therapy, and specifically group analytic therapy, it has applications across all modalities of psychodynamic therapy. The unequivocal message is that all trainings, theories, and practices of therapy are not fit for purpose in a racist world without intersectionality. The provocations of this book, born out of lived experience, are necessarily unapologetic, disruptive, transgressive, and explicitly direct. For example, Farideh Dizadji asks, 'I am now wondering by submission of this published conversation, whether I can allow myself to 'to be exposed', to 'join in', 'to become part of', 'to accept my own differences and the intersectionality of my multiple identities'? And finally, 'where do I choose to position myself or and belong to? I am a political refugee in exile since 1984. It seems there are correlations between working through my trauma caused by state organized violence, and my personal journey within the context of power, position, and privilege, which have been evolving over the years'. Reem Shelhi states in Chapter 4 of this book,

> Crenshaw's metaphor of 'traffic' invokes for me neither flow nor congestion, but the mangled cold metallic wreckage of a crash site. This pileup of twisted parts, half, never whole, and yet too much, intimates not only the contours of gender, the skin of ethnicity, the mouth of sexuality and the eyes of shame, but also entangled and intangible clusters, including forms of privilege. The complexity of my contextually kaleidoscopic identity means that themes are so interlinked, that one cannot be mentioned without another being inferred, and yet another throwing the next off course.

Reem Shelhi concludes, 'my work continues, unpicking the knots of injured intersectionality one stitch at a time, and learning to stand – upright and embodied – in my own power'. Suryia Nayak recalls in Chapter 5 of this book,

> *My parents shared a migratory experience of moving from homelands subjected to colonialism. They shared the common experience of 'No Irish, No Blacks, No dogs.' I was born into an intergenerational social unconscious of colonialism*

DOI: 10.4324/9781003232216-1

and racism. I have carried this my whole life . . . My group analytic journey has enabled me to see the malignant mirroring of 'No Irish, No Blacks, No dogs' in group therapy, supervision, and large group experiences.

The profound messages and learning of this book are because the authors believe that 'silence will not protect' (Lorde, 1977:41). The courage and risks that the authors of this edited collection have taken in writing their chapters are testimony to the fact that intersectionality is a method of transforming silence into language and action (ibid.). To read is to bear witness. No longer ignorant of intersectionality, the question is, what are you going to do beyond testimony and witness?

This edited collection forms a group of positions relating to a common concern of the interdependency of difference. Like the experience of being in a group, the intersection of different perspectives in this book produces something greater than the sum of the individual perspectives. True to the idea that content and method are co-productive, the group analytic content of this book grew out of a group process method. The process of writing this book was deliberately held through group processes of authors meeting collectively at different times and in different configurations to reflect on the development of their ideas. The organic evolution of this book reflects the organic growth of a group process.

This book is for people who are new to the idea of intersectionality and for those who are searching for new ways of putting intersectionality to work. Examples of new iterations of intersectionality developed in this book include Anne Aiyegbusi's 'intersectional matrix'; Anthea Benjamin's 'intersectional consciousness', 'empathic intersectionality' and 'intersectional language'; Daniel Anderson's 'group polyphony' and 'location of difference'; and Reem Shelhi's 'Affectivism' and 'locations of discovery'.

The big questions are:

- How does your therapeutic practice work with difference?
- No one's identity and context are ever made up of a single factor such as race, sexuality, gender, class, or disability. How does your therapeutic practice work with the crisscrossing of simultaneous multiple differences?
- How does your therapeutic practice explicitly address the trauma of overlapping oppressive social constructions?

The importance of anti-racist feminist theoretical frames in group therapy, psychotherapy, and counselling is becoming increasingly recognized as relevant to equity of service provision, training, and research (see Group Analysis Special Issue on Racism, 2021: vol. 54, 3). Putting intersectionality to work recognizes

intersectionality's transformative potentials are a license to experiment with new approaches to psychotherapy training and practice that take a radical approach to human cultural diversity that rejects the easy buzzwords of 'diversity,' 'inclusion,' and 'intersecting identities' and embraces the challenging discourse of power, inequality, and justice.

(Grzanka, 2020:244)

This book directly addresses the relationship between the Black feminist concept of intersectionality and group analysis as a form of group therapy (with transferable relevance to diverse modes of group therapy). One of the most significant contributions that intersectionality offers Group Analysis is a sustained focus on the inextricable interdependencies of power, privilege, and position. Scholz explains the importance of exposing these interconnections:

power [is] an integral element of all human relationships and any social order. . . . And discussing power at the same time means discussing privileges. Invisibility and unconsciousness of power consequently means invisibility of privileges, which makes them well-protected.

(Scholz, 2004:527–528)

Putting intersectionality to work sustains a theoretical emphasis as a scaffolding for clinical experience to enable discourses of power, position, and privilege in Group Analysis and psychodynamic therapeutic approaches to be developed. The non-divisible clinical-political imperative for therapeutic intersectionality rests on the fact that 'systems of segregation, ghettoization or colonization are replicated in analytic groups' (Aiyegbusi, 2021a, 2021b).

This book responds to the urgency for the development of clinically relevant theory to enable group analysis to be fit for purpose in an intersectionally racist landscape. Black Lives Matter and the ongoing implications of the global pandemic of Covid-19 continue to expose existing structural inequalities that provoke an urgency within Group Analysis to include theories of liberation such as Black feminism and other anti-racist, anti-colonial conceptual frameworks.

The work in this edited collection is grounded in clinical practice and lived experiences and responds to questions such as:

- How does intersectionality enable anti-racist therapeutic group work that is equipped to consider, for example, the compound injuries of class and sexuality?
- How do theoretical exchanges between intersectionality, and modalities of psychotherapy, including Group Analysis, contribute to explorations of inevitable issues of power, position, and privilege in group-analytic training, practice, and organization?
- Does the relationship between intersectionality and Group Analysis demonstrate the necessity for Group Analysis to allow its slow, open theoretical group to accommodate outsider concepts?

The metanarrative of this book calls for the 'decolonizing' of group analytic training, therapeutic practice, and institutional traditions. The call for anti-racist, anti-colonial Group Analysis is fraught with tensions because all institutes, discourses, and social constructions are 'implicated', occupying 'an ambiguous position' within oppressive structures (Caselli, 2005:105). However, Group Analysis is a mechanism and movement for reparation and transformation, and therefore, the imperative is to grapple with Azu-Okeke's question of 'whether, given the ethos of group analysis, we can accommodate the interests of all who are affected by the consequences of colonialism' (2003:476).

What Is Intersectionality?

An intersection is a place where two or more roads cross or meet. Nayak explains, 'Intersectionality is a metaphor that uses the idea of a crossroads to think about the injury of being hit by the crash of multiple vehicles of oppression travelling on different roads of social inequality' (Crenshaw, 1989:149). There is never a quiet moment on the roads of social inequality, and the number, design, and function of the vehicles never cease. Furthermore, these are reckless vehicles bound for collision. The point is that being in the intersection means inevitable injury. For example, a Black working-class woman living at the intersection of race, class, and gender will suffer the compound impact of being simultaneously hit by the oppression of racism, patriarchy, and class inequality. Conversely, intersectionality can be used to think about the protection and advantages of multiple privileges of whiteness, heterosexuality, patriarchy, and capitalism. In this frame, the metaphorical possibilities of the crossroads may include 'the absence of cars, or perhaps the absence of the road altogether' (Rodó-Zárate and Jorba, 2022:25). The point is that situated positionality in the intersection of power and privilege is a complex configuration. Intersectionality provides an analytic lens on the compound injury of oppression, while enabling analysis of the compound effects of social advantage (Nayak, 2022:327).

Psychotherapy is concerned with psychological injury, and intersectionality is a psychosocial lens on compound injury caused by abuses of power – note the plural. No act or experience of subjugation and silencing is ever singular. Abuse of power does not function in splendid isolation. Abuse of power, the use of power over people, always depends upon and is contingent upon other axes of abuses of power and power over. Avtar Brah explains that abuses of power 'cannot be treated as "independent variables", because the oppression of each is inscribed within the other – is constituted by, and is constitutive of the other' (Brah, 1996:109). Intersectionality names and frames how different forms of oppression are mutually constitutive of each other – herein lies intersectionality's therapeutic power of reparative healing.

Although the word intersectionality was coined by the critical race legal scholar Kimberlé Crenshaw in 1989, the historical roots of intersectionality (Ilmonen, 2019) lie in the struggles of Black women who knew from their lived experience of multiple oppression that focusing on either race or gender or socio-economic inequality was simply inadequate and (re)produces oppression (Alarcón, 1990; Anzaldúa, 2007; Cooper, 2017 [1982]; Brah and Phoenix, 2004; Cade Bambara,

2005; Christian, 1987; Bhavnani, 2001; Davis, 1981; Hill Collins, 2000; Hull et al., 1982; Lorde, 1984; Mohanty, 2003; Phoenix and Pattynama, 2006; The Combahee River Collective, 1977; Truth, 1851; Walker, 1982). Crenshaw explains that

> *the intersection of racism and sexism factors into Black women's lives in ways that cannot be captured wholly by looking at the race or gender dimensions of those experiences separately . . . the intersections of race and gender highlights the need to account for multiple grounds of identity when considering how the social world is constructed.*
>
> (Crenshaw, 1991:1244–1245)

The problem is that the social world is constructed along the lines of divisions, demarcations, and categories precisely designed to manage multiplicity, especially interconnected interdependent multiplicity. Meanwhile, human experience does not fit into separate, distinct lines of divisions, demarcations, and categories. Indeed, divisions, demarcations, and categories constitute the experience of trauma. Paradoxically, but not by coincidence, a frequent response to trauma is to put the distress into a mental box in an effort to demarcate and separate trauma from day-to-day living. Nayak explains that:

> *Fragmentation, division, and disconnection are traumatic and also form false ineffective coping mechanisms for alienation and marginalisation. However, perversely most of us unconsciously use fragmentation and disconnection to work with fragmentation and disconnection (Chantler, 2005). Disconnection is a tool of oppression and, more specifically, a tool of racism. To complicate matters further, racism is always interconnected to other vectors of oppression. Racism functions through a double bind of interconnection and disconnection using interconnection via capillary webs of power (Foucault, 1980) and disconnection to distract and disempower discernment of its machinations. The insidious force of this internalised backdrop explains why we have to work hard to unlearn 'dividing practices' (Foucault, 1975; 1993 [1982]) and why intersectionality, which is based on a simple metaphor of an intersection, is feared, resisted, and misunderstood.*
>
> (Nayak, 2022:325)

Furthermore, the social world constructs identity categories in hierarchical ranking where some identities and contexts are given more power, privilege, and position, and some identities and contexts are marginalized, subjugated, silenced, and abjected. Social world constructions have a habit of becoming internal world constructions. The lived experience of being in the intersection of numerous simultaneous social constructions of oppression has a corresponding intersectional psychological impact, and that impact is injurious and traumatic. Any group analytic or psychotherapy framework, theory or mode of practice that does not address the compound effect of being hit at the crossroads by the collision of multiple oppression is not fit for purpose. Group Analysis and modalities of psychotherapy could take heed from the analogies that Crenshaw used,

> *analogous to a doctor's decision at the scene of an accident to treat an accident victim only if the injury is recognized by medical insurance. Similarly, providing legal relief only when Black women show that their claims are based on race or on sex is analogous to calling an ambulance for the victim only after the driver responsible for the injuries is identified. But it is not always easy to reconstruct an accident: Sometimes the skid marks and the injuries simply indicate that they occurred simultaneously, frustrating efforts to determine which driver caused the harm. In these cases, the tendency seems to be that no driver is held responsible, no treatment is administered, and the involved parties simply get back in their cars and zoom away.*
>
> (Crenshaw, 1989:149)

These questions arise:

- Do Group Analysis and other modalities of dynamic therapy only work with psychic injuries or wounds from configurations of collisions recognized by their manuals (external and internal texts)?
- How do Group Analysis and other modalities of dynamic therapy enable a reconstruction of the psychic collision of multiple oppression?
- Working across differences of power, privilege, and position, how are unconscious transference and countertransference communications worked through when the psychotherapist or group therapy conductor is actually or symbolically representative of the driver causing the injury?

In this book, Aiyegbusi's chapter talks about the importance of 'intersectional preparation' of group therapy co-conductors. Aiyegbusi states in Chapter 1,

> *as a result of their preparation, Dr Adebanjo and Mr James were able to respect each other's personal intersectional matrices and were able to learn about the multi-dimensional ways their intersecting axes of identity manifest in the social world and consider the probable interactions with others' intersectional matrices within a group context.*

It is ethically incumbent on group analytic and psychotherapy trainings, theories, practice, and supervision to hold an intersectional lens (Nayak, 2020a). Not to do so, returning to Crenshaw's analogy, is the equivalent of getting 'back in their cars and zoom[ing] away'.

Crenshaw used a traffic crossroads to explain that 'intersectional experience is greater than the sum of racism and sexism' (Crenshaw, 1989:140). However, others have used different metaphors (Rodó-Zárate and Jorba, 2022) to show how and why the intermixture of different forms of oppression produces something greater than an addition or subtraction formula such as one plus one plus one type of equations or framings. Simply naming the vehicles of oppression along different roads of social inequality is not intersectionality. Simply stating that there are multiple forms of oppression or counting numerous directions of social inequality is not intersectionality.

Putting intersectionality to work rejects addition and subtraction formula approaches to widening participation (increasing diversity and inclusion through additional numbers/skin pigmentation) because 'problems of exclusion cannot be solved simply by including Black [people] within an already established analytical structure' (Crenshaw, 1989:140). Thus, the conditions of a theoretical reciprocity between Group Analysis and intersectionality mean more than being added to a reference list, inclusion in citations, and being the subject of a special issue or lecture/workshop. This point is taken up in this book by Claire Bacha and Dick Blackwell, where Blackwell states in Chapter 7,

> *putting Kimberlé Crenshaw, bell hooks and Angela Davis, and indeed Suryia Nayak and Anne Aiyegbusi, on a reading list doesn't go very far if they're going to be taught in the same authoritarian way and examined through dissertations marked by politburo panels of readers, who probably know less than the students.*

Whether in the interpersonal encounters of individual psychotherapy or the transpersonal dynamics of group psychotherapy, the intersectional experience of race, class, gender, sexuality, age, and other socio-economic factors run simultaneously in multiple directions, enacting configuration of power, privilege, and position. Intersectionality rests on the 'greater than' compound effect. Ken (2008) uses a culinary metaphor:

> *Because the cookie's flavor is constructed as it collides with the tongue, the possibility exists that each tongue may experience it differently. Like sugar, butter, eggs, and flour, which do not simply "interlock" or "intersect," combinations of race, class, and gender intermingle like flavors in our mouths. We taste them. We experience them. Race, class, and gender's meanings transform when they come in contact with those who taste them, who enact them, who need them, who rely on them, who hate them, who are oppressed by them, who get advantages from them, who do not realize they are there, who do them, who use them. Undoubtedly, this means these combinations end up with many different meanings.*
> (Ken, 2008:164)

Particularly useful for Group Analysis, Ken's culinary metaphor brings the relational, visceral, embodied experience of intersectionality to life. In this book, Benjamin's chapter on Black Women's Bodies draws on clinical practice to illustrate that

> *oppression and discrimination affect how we view both ourselves and the bodies we are in, it lodges in our system, skin, flesh, and bones. This becomes a form of trauma that is all too often dismissed. Bodies that are positioned as*

non-normative identities experience significant traumatic effects which lead to profound experiences of projection and disembodiment which need naming and addressing.

In the context of racialized misogyny, the psychic defence of expressing trauma via the body through somatization to survive the embodied experience of the compound injuries of racism and patriarchy necessitates psychotherapeutic intersectional formulations of somatization. In short, theatres of the body are intersectional (Nayak, 2021b:524). Translated to the practice of group therapy and Group Analysis, the following question highlights tensions that need intersectional supervisory support: 'What are the implications for the group matrix, where a patient and/or group conductor brings the "intersectional experience of being the Black daughter of white mother, and/or white mother who maybe overtly racist" (Nayak, 2020b:456).

Intersectionality advocates that intersecting axes of power and difference, which operate simultaneously to (re)inscribe marginality and privilege, cannot be 'layered onto each other in an additive or hierarchical way' (Mirza and Gunaratnam, 2014:128). As an anti-border theory, intersectionality problematizes fixed, theoretical, and disciplinary divisions. In short, intersectionality provides an argument for resistance to the split between theory and practice, centre, and margin, individual and collective, subject and context, mind/body, and paternalistic service provider/ professional and service recipient/user binary relations. Intersectionality's contestation of fragmentation and borders enables thinking and practice with the mutually constitutive 'multidimensionality' of experience and practice and refuses a 'single-axis' analysis.

The primary task of putting intersectionality to work in therapeutic practice, including clinical supervision, reflective discussions, and recording of clinical work, is to understand the interdependent interconnections of oppression. This requires an understanding of the meaning of interdependency and the meaning of interconnection. Putting intersectionality to work is to articulate how the interdependency or mutually constitutive relationship of links in the chain of power produces something greater than simply naming the links in the chain. In group analytic therapy, putting intersectionality to work includes consciously mapping the intersections of location and directional forces of oppression within the dynamics of the group (Nayak, 2022). The group conductor should enable the naming and analysis of macro and micro aggressions of oppression and their compound injury as they inevitably manifest in the group. The framework of putting intersectionality to work by Nayak (2022) proposes four tasks to prompt intersectional thinking and hold in mind conscious and unconscious intersectional dynamics:

- Name the roads of social inequality and how they crisscross.
- Name the vehicles of oppression on roads of social inequality.
- Describe the crash/collision at the intersection.
- Describe the bio-psycho-social injuries.

Name the Roads of Social Inequality and How They Crisscross

Naming the roads of social inequality locates issues within macro social structures. This prompts the identification (through naming) and contextualisation (through situating or locating) of the issues under examination. Mapping the cartography of the roads of social inequality restrains the myopic gaze on the individual, family and/or community that uncouples the presenting problem embodied by the individual, family and/or community from broader forces of power. Naming the roads of social inequality situates the problem in the contexts that people inhabit, rather than the habits of people.

(Nayak, 2022:328)

Name the Vehicles of Oppression on Roads of Social Inequality

The vehicles on the roads of social inequality are the mechanisms that drive oppression and discrimination (social constructions, discourses, attitudes, and behaviours). Vehicles of oppression travel in multiple directions and come in multiple guises or design versions (juggernauts, trucks, cars, motorbikes and so on). The task is to name the vehicles of oppression that are hitting the person(s) at the intersection. This prompts granular analysis of the specificity of different forms of oppression, while building a picture of the compound severity of being simultaneously hit by multiple forces of power. Naming the vehicles of oppression hitting the person(s) in the intersections of their lives develops the detail of the contextual picture of power that people inhabit, thereby reducing the tendency to see the issues that people bring as an inherent impairment or dysfunction of their personality. It enables increased understanding of the complexity of the lived experience of power.

(Nayak, 2022:329)

Describe the Crash/Collision at the Intersection

Analysis of the crash exposes why and how vehicles of oppression are reckless. Dangerous driving, correspond to the recklessness of oppression (road rage, intoxication, moving too fast/slow, distraction, exhaustion, carelessness, entitlement, distorted perspective). Reckless driving in group analytic therapy and all modalities of psychotherapy might include the distorted perspective and behaviours of white privilege, heteronormativity, class privilege and entitlement; the distraction of bureaucracy and commodification; the exhaustion of the intensification of work; the road rage (conscious and unconscious) of people not conforming to professional expert knowledge or ethnocentric orders of discourse; and the intoxication of confirmation bias. Not resting with the naming of the roads and vehicles of subjugation, the task is to drill down to understand the modus operandi of different vehicles of oppression. The task is to build a picture of the compound impact of multiple methods of power colliding simultaneously in the lives of people. It is a task of moving from generalities to specificity that sharpens practices of active listening to the situated knowledge of lived experience by heightening alertness to the specificity of intersecting modus operandi of oppression. For example, the distinct idiosyncrasies of how racism, sexism and homophobia are experienced in the particular life of individuals, families and communities will differ from one context to another. Moving from a generalised picture to a particularised picture of the compound impact of multiple methods of racist oppression mitigates the imposition of cultural competency.

(Nayak, 2022:330)

Describe the Bio-psycho-social Injuries

By now, a detailed contextual picture of the multiple intersecting complexities of the situation or context of oppression for an individual or group is developing. The function of understanding the injury at the intersection of colliding reckless vehicles of oppression is to reposition shame, blame, pathology, and stigma from people to the contexts and impacts of oppression. For example, the weathering effect of intersectional racism recognises the individual subjective reality of the biological, psychological, and social harm of depression, alopecia, high blood pressure, alcoholism and social anxiety, while locating the systemic cause in racist social structures.

(Ibid.)

For clinicians undertaking research, Winker and Degele (2011) propose putting intersectionality to work using a model of intersectional analysis in eight steps that are particularly useful for facilitating the analysis of the empirical material.

Intersectionality and Group Analytic Theory

Intersectionality could be explained through the simile that Foulkes (the founder of group analysis) uses to describe the relational process of Group Analysis:

> *suppose you have to wash a number of dirty shirts together, and the water is not even clean and perhaps you have not even soap . . . even then you can get the shirts reasonably clean, albeit you add dirt to dirt, by using them for mutual friction upon each other.*

(Foulkes, 1948:29)

Dirty shirts and dirt could be understood as the psychic disturbance of the intersectional effects of the social conditioning of disconnection and marginalization. Here, the group analytic situation as a space where the collective 'mutual friction' of individual member's disturbance is transformed would attend to how we are all 'constrained by social events' (Hopper, 1982:153) of fragmentation (re)produced in and through oppression (Pines, 2014). Intersectionality enables analysis of processes of disconnection and intersection that foreground power. Tubert-Oklander asks that Group Analysis be thought of as 'an interdisciplinary enterprise ... through an open dialogue with its peers in the field of human thought' (2019:422). Such a 'peer in the field' is intersectionality. Intersectionality is an effective tool for the analysis of interdependency, interconnectedness, hybridity plurality, and simultaneity (Crenshaw, 2017; Cho et al., 2013; Fotopoulou, 2012; Grzanka, 2014; McCall, 2005; McKinnon, 2013; Nayak, 2021; Purkayastha, 2012; Yuval-Davis, 2014). Moreover, intersectionality questions the separation of the inseparable (Gunnarsson, 2017). These characteristics are core to the theoretical basis and practice of Group Analysis, conveyed in the shape of a circle to 'allow every member to see every other member ... where everybody is equal' (Foulkes, 1975:81); and in the idea that the experience of the group is greater than the sum of its individual members. Group Analysis and intersectionality share the following characteristics, as described by Dalal (1998:39):

1 The 'part' is always connected to the 'whole'.
2 The 'whole' determines what takes place in the 'parts'.
3 The 'whole' is always an artefact, an abstraction that is carved out of a greater complexity.

Elias's focus on the principle of interdependency is captured in the following analogy, 'we say the wind is blowing, as if the wind were separate from its blowing, as if a wind could exist which did not blow' (Elias, 1999:112). Lavie (2005:522–525) uses a conversation between Brown and Elias (Brown, 1997:518–519) to demonstrate the 'Simultaneous-Interdependent Process of "Individualization" and "Socialization": The First Root of Group-Analytic Theory'. This title describes a process that is at the root of intersectionality. Furthermore, the foundational group-analytic concept of figuration where 'the constituent parts is identical ... to the composite unit' (Elias, 1978:176; Dalal, 2001:88–90) is also foundational to intersectionality. In the following statement, Razack proposes a constitutive symbiosis between the intersecting systems that produce particular positions:

> *Interlocking systems need one another, and in tracing the complex ways in which they help to secure one another, we learn how women are produced into positions that exist symbiotically but hierarchically.*
>
> (Razack, 1998:13)

In group-analytic terms, it could be argued that Razack (who is not a group analyst) points to the relational 'tracing' process of group analytic practice. Furthermore, because the 'word position has the advantage of being at once relational and spatial' (Liveras, 2020:9), Razack's foregrounding of the idea that intersecting contexts produce intersecting positionalities resonates with group-analytic understandings of 'relational processes as "co-constructed" rather than "projected" or "introjected"' (Liveras, 2020:29). In this frame, Razack's Black feminist intersectional theorizing has congruence with Liveras's group analytic 'language of positioning in figurations' (ibid.). Moreover, Razack's inclusion of hierarchy brings the issue of unequal power relations into the frame.

Contextual Intersectionality and Group Analysis

The importance of context, location, and situatedness is reiterated across the different perspectives in this book. Under the lens of intersectionality, the group analytical concept of 'the location of disturbance' is seen from different angles that theoretically develop the idea of the location of disturbance. Examples of putting intersectionality to work on the group analytic concept of location include Anderson's chapter, which argues for the move from the 'location of disturbance' to 'location of difference'; Shelhi's chapter, which argues for a transformation of 'locations of disturbance' into 'locations of discovery'; and Dizadji and Nayak's chapter which stresses the imperative of 'Locational intersectionality' stating,

> *Over and over again the issue of location appears central to intersectionality and more specifically to an intersectional articulation of the trauma of being a political refugee. An intersectional group therapy approach to the location of disturbance opens curiosity of location as a multiple undecidable situation.*

The group analyst Earl Hopper goes to the etymology of the word 'context' to demonstrate a discursive lineage where the

> *prefix coil is related to cum, meaning "together", "together with", "in combination" and "in union" . . . the stem word "text" has . . . two elementary but interdependent roots. The first, textus, means "tissue". . . . The second root is texere, meaning "to weave".*

(Hopper, 1982:138)

Connotations of the coming 'together' of the 'weave' of multiple lived experience enables appreciation of the importance of context in the theory and practice of Group Analysis, which is shared by the theory and practice of intersectionality. Hopper explains that

> *in order to understand the transference, it must be contextualized, that is, related to other categories of events which stand in specified relationships to the transference in terms of time and social psychological space.*

(Hopper, 1982:139)

The implications for understanding transference as contextualized in power can be seen in Probyn's statement that 'the space and place we inhabit produce us' (2003:294). Using Probyn's logic, in terms of the transformative potential of Group Analysis, it follows that inhabiting the space and place of the analytic group will produce a different 'us'. The tension is that whilst a group may create an 'alternative belief system' (Garland, 2010:215), the group-analytic situation will always be a microcosm of wider socio-political dynamics of power. The special issue of Group Analysis on the implications of 'Contemporary Social Theory' for Group Analysis highlights the importance of the 'process or context in which such identifications happen [and] the arenas of activity that enable or constrain the affirmation of particular allegiances or designations' (Burman and Frosh, 2005:10). This edited collection demonstrates that the social theory of intersectionality brings the issue of power within intersubjective social relations into sharp focus. In this frame, there is nothing neutral about Group Analysis.

In terms of context, Black feminists speak of the 'politics of location' (Boyce Davies, 1994:153), where the power dynamics (politics) of location function simultaneously as the 'what' and the 'how' of social relations. The anti-colonial scholar Radhakrishnan argues that

The politics of location is productive . . . it makes one location vulnerable to the claims of another and enables multiple contested readings of the one reality from a variety of locations and positions.

(2000:56–57)

Radhakrishnan's analysis is congruent with Foulkes' insistence on location as a dynamic 'process' (Foulkes, 1986:131). This dynamic process troubles demarcations of the beginning and end of what is inside and outside a border. The implications can be highly anxiety-provoking, in terms of being 'vulnerable' to the 'Other', whether that is an internalized 'Other' within self or the 'Other' within the dynamics of interpersonal therapeutic relationships. In this frame, the 'location' of each 'disturbance' (Foulkes, 1990:184) is also the disturbing location of the 'Other' and this is a matter of power.

If identity, subjectivity, and psychological distress are a product of the intersectional racist conditions and contexts people inhabit, then,

[t]he problems of madness and misery, then, lie not inevitably in any inherent impairment of perception, emotion or conduct. . . . Instead, they are located in the contexts they inhabit.

(Pilgrim and Rogers, 2008:36)

This resonates with Foulkes' theory that each person is an 'abstraction' of the contexts they inhabit or 'basically and centrally determined, inevitably, by the world in which he lives, by the community, the group, of which he forms a part' (Foulkes, 1948:10; see also Pichon-Rivière, 1979:57). Likewise, intersectionality emphasizes context as the producer of identity but places increased emphasis on the constitution of difference within unequal power relations. For example, Anthias argues that 'forms of social distinction and inequality are produced in complex combinatories of social location' (2011:214). Exemplified through intersectionality, the significance of context is central to Black feminist theory, where the concept of location moves from being a noun to a verb or method to trouble location as space (Nayak, 2017). This is apparent in Crenshaw's choice of the word 'mapping' (1991), Huggan's 'cartographic connections' (1989:128), Boyce Davies' 'compasses of racialization' (2013:173–201), Mohanty's 'cartographies of struggle' (2003), and Brah's 'Cartographies of Diaspora' (1996). Minh-ha states that 'if you can't locate the other, how are you going to locate yourself?' (Minh-ha, 1991:73).

The complexity of locating self and others within Group Analytic experience is articulated by Weegmann in the following question, 'how does one describe a landscape, without already being part of it? (2014:58). The complexity of Weegmann's question is amplified when the 'colossal forces' (Foulkes, 1964:52) of social constraints of 'intolerant norms and the fetish for rationality' (Pilgrim and Rogers, 2008:36) are brought into the equation. Furthermore, as Shelhi's biographical chapter in this book so directly testifies, within the landscape of intersectional racism, social constraints constitute the terms of who and what is welcomed and attended to in group therapy and training. In refusing intolerant norms of fragmented identity categories, intersectionality enables a nuanced tracking of multiple simultaneous intersections of power (re)produced in the 'landscape' of the social. From a group-analytic perspective, Dalal summarizes the challenge,

[t]he problem is that it is much easier to visualize a unitary particle, and nigh impossible to visualize a field. A particle, an individual, is bounded and looks infinite to the eye. This makes it easier for us to formulate thoughts about it, relate it to other things. . . . In contrast a field is so much more amorphous, it is fluctuating continuum with no end in sight.

(Dalal, 1998:221)

Temporal Interconnections in Intersectionality and Group Analysis

In this book, the chapter by Dizadji and Nayak on an intersectional understanding of trauma experienced by political refugees argues for nuanced attention to the function of time in the experience and context of extreme trauma. The call is to attend to the temporal dimensions of intersectionality. Here, putting intersectionality to work sharpens the focus on positionalities of identity and context to include analysis of the forces of time, the historical, intergenerational aspects of the production of subjectivity and situated knowledge. The group analyst Hopper explains that

I try to explore a fuller range of events on the dimensions of time and social psychological space . . . I would like to remind you that even Dr. Bion did not give us much guidance on how to apply his cryptic statement – which is in effect the starting point of my thinking – that the "basic assumption group knows no time.

(1982:140)

It could be said that the experience of intersectionality 'knows no time' and has congruence with Hopper's (1997) 'Fourth Basic Assumption'. Although 1989 is identified as the date when the word 'intersectionality' was coined by Crenshaw, the concept of intersectionality is founded upon an indeterminate historical legacy of Black feminist struggles. Brah and Phoenix base their analysis of intersectionality on the 1851 speech entitled 'Ain't I a Woman' by the slave woman Sojourner Truth:

> *[W]e begin this paper with the 19th century political locution 'Ain't I a Woman?' precisely because . . . it neatly captures all the main elements of the debate on 'intersectionality'. We regard the concept of 'intersectionality' as signifying the complex, irreducible, varied, and variable effects which ensue when multiple axis of differentiation – economic, political, cultural, psychic, subjective and experiential – intersect in historically specific contexts.*
>
> (Brah and Phoenix, 2004:76)

The Combahee River Collective was a 'radical Black feminist organization formed in 1974 and named after Harriet Tubman's 1853 raid on the Combahee River in South Carolina that freed 750 enslaved people' (Taylor, 2017:4), and their 'Statement' (1977) of purpose describes why a temporal situated intersectional lens on their experience was important,

> *The most general statement of our politics at the present time . . . [is] the development of integrated analysis and practice based upon the fact that the major systems of oppression or are interlocking. The synthesis of these oppressions creates the conditions of our lives.*
>
> (The Combahee River Collective, 1977:261)

The Combahee Collective's reference to 'present time', 'systems', and 'conditions' places emphasis on temporal situated context, indicating that processes of subjectification cannot be divorced from circumstances. The Combahee Collective's assertion that the 'synthesis of . . . oppressions creates the conditions of our lives' resonates with Foulkes' notion of the 'process of configurational analysis as the "location" of each disturbance' (1990:184). Intersectionality enables analysis of the 'disturbance' of intersectional experiences in the 'location' of 'racial, sexual, heterosexual, and class oppression' (The Combahee River Collective, 1977:261) functioning through active configurations of relational communication networks on simultaneous multiple levels of interpersonal dynamics. The name 'Combahee Collective' signifies a historical consciousness or intergenerational legacy from over a century prior to the formation of the collective – which, in keeping with the spirit of Group Analysis, operated according to democratic group structure principles (Nitzgen, 2001). Just as early developmental roots are an important feature in understanding the evolution and development of group-analytic theory and are foundational to group analytic practice (Raufman and Weinberg, 2016), temporal interconnections with the historical roots of Black feminism were important for The Combahee Collective, and this remains the case for the evolution Black feminist theory, including intersectionality. Intersectionality is a product of the 'trans-generational transmission' (Hopper and Weinberg, 2011) of Black women's intersectional experiences forged within the temporal social unconscious (Biran, 2014; Hopper, 2003; Weinberg, 2007) of racism (Blackwell, 2014). Perhaps what Group Analysis offers intersectionality is a theory of how the 'the social [is] integral to the unconscious [and], the unconscious is constituted by the social at *every* level' (Dalal, 2001:554, emphasis in original). A reciprocal theoretical exchange between intersectionality and Group Analysis would provide an understanding of how socially constructed divisions of difference function as conscious structural and unconscious 'groupal' (Knauss, 2006:163) processes. Intersectionality and Group Analysis both 'attempt to illuminate the historical matrix' (Davis, 1971) of experience. Whilst the resonances between Group Analysis and intersectionality continue to emerge, offering a basis for a theoretical exchange, the real test is in living together.

The social unconscious, configured and contingent upon temporal interconnections, acquires a traumatic characteristic in the abuse of power. Blackwell points out that '[t]he colonial patterns of relationship remain deep in our social unconscious' (2003:456). The temporal dimension of Hopper's (1997) 'Fourth Basic Assumption' enables understanding of how intergenerational trauma is performatively (re)produced (Butler, 1997, 1999) in the social unconscious of traumatized societies through oscillating polarities of aggregation and massification. Theoretical reciprocity between Hopper's oeuvre on trauma, the social unconscious, and the fourth basic assumption with anti-racist, Post-colonial, Critical Race, and Black feminist oeuvres would enhance the practice of therapeutic groups where oscillating polarities of assimilation and alienation (Treacher, 2005) are communicated through dynamics such as transference, projective identification, and countertransference (Milivojevic, 2005). Weinberg states that

> *[t]his theme is definitely a deep Social Unconscious issue transmitted over generations in a society of immigrants, affecting the way different ethnic groups integrate in this multicultural society. . . . The Social Unconscious reveals itself also in traumatized societies and in community and national crisis events.*
>
> (2007:318)

In the context of globalization, applications of Group Analysis that extend 'beyond clinical theory and method' (Rohr, 2014:367) are needed. In this book, Dizadji and Nayak's chapter on an intersectional response to the intersectionality of trauma demonstrates the challenges for group-analytics with traumatized refugees and asylum seekers (Rohr, 2018; Tucker, 2011). A mutually constitutive theoretical exchange between the temporal interconnections in intersectionality and Group Analysis would enable group therapy practitioners to understand that

> *group events (why patients behave as they do) are understood through the transference by reference to past history, and the history that is used is the history of*

asocial individuals. . . . [This] throws into relief the absence of a group-analytic
paradigm, one that might take account of the history of social groups.

(Dalal, 1998:12–13)

Structure of the Book

Anne Aiyegbusi's chapter 'Holding the Broken Pieces: An Intersectional Approach
to Group Analysis for Women in Prison' argues that intersectionality is particularly
relevant for group work with women of colour who are incarcerated because intersectionality is

- A framework offering the analytic capacity to understand the impact of multiple
  marginalized identities.
- Rooted in the lived experience of socially and politically oppressed and voiceless persons.
- Committed to holding together and integrating all the parts of a person or community that have become fragmented with many labels, borders, and divisions.

In Chapter 1, Aiyegbusi points to the 'pressure to try to convert complexity into
simplicity may feel overwhelming, mirroring the women's internal struggles with
uncontainable and typically unfathomable emotional experiences'. Aiyegbusi
coins the term 'intersectional matrix' to 'capture the interaction of multiple facets
of identity and the way these emerge and play out within the matrix of an analytic
group'. Aiyegbusi puts the idea of the 'intersectional matrix' to work to 'capture
the impact, interplay and complexity involved in containing and working analytically with a considerable range and multiplicity of stigmatised and marginalised
identities and the intensity of associated trauma, including that which became
criminogenic'. Aiyegbusi asserts that holding the 'intersectional matrix' in therapeutic group work

> *emphasises a focus on difference and the interaction within the matrix of*
> *both complimentary and conflicting identities. It highlights the depth of*
> *thought afforded to oppression trauma and its replication within the group*
> *matrix, including as offence paralleling behaviour. The term intersectional*
> *matrix also aims to draw attention to the empirical knowledge of an oth-*
> *erwise voiceless population and the intention of group process to mobilise*
> *its members' agency with regard to establishing a shared narrative which*
> *is rooted in their lived experience, and which serves to co-create a robust*
> *dynamic matrix.*

Anthea Benjamin's chapter, 'Do Black Women's Bodies Matter in Group Analysis? Moving from double to intersectional consciousness' introduces the new concepts of 'critical intersectional consciousness' and 'empathic intersectionality' to
enable an intersectional language of communication required to address the needs

of black women. Benjamin challenges colonial patriarchal roots and tools of psychoanalytic frameworks, stating in Chapter 2,

> *[This is] the precise problem that Audre Lorde makes reference to in her question, What does it mean when the tools of a racist patriarchy are used to examine the fruits of that same patriarchy?' Lorde's answer is, 'It means that only the narrowest perimeters of change are possible and allowable' which points to the process of (re)enactment.*

Benjamin moves from Du Bois' idea of 'double consciousness' to 'intersectional consciousness'. Benjamin's chapter insists that

> *the group conductor needs to have done and to continue to do their own work on their own intersectional identities, as the group as a whole will be reflecting the conductor's own fragmentation. This is because groups reflect the conductor's own unprocessed and processed parts of their psyche. It is here where we can expand the frame beyond the master's tools so that we can better address the historical and ongoing harm being done to the marginalised bodies of Black women.*

Daniel Anderson's chapter 'The Body of the Group: Sexuality, Transgender, and Group Polyphony' uses the 1970 film *The Boys in the Band* and clinical vignette material to produce an intersectional queer analysis of sexuality and (trans)gender in relation to group analysis. In Chapter 3, Anderson contends that 'group analysis has failed to fully articulate the sexual and gender minorities beyond heteronormativity and psychopathology'. Anderson argues that 'Much has been written about the apparently pathological nature of the 'homosexual'. Very little has turned this around to consider the pathology-inducing nature of the discourse within certain schools of psychoanalysis surrounding the 'homosexual' and the 'pervert' that subsequently results in traumatizing the subject. The prolific nature of such writings and their pervasive existence within Western society at least has become akin to a 'death by a thousand cuts'. Anderson introduces the term 'group polyphony' to 'disrupt positions of power and privilege by recognising the equality of voices within the group where the political and apolitical intersect'. Anderson argues for a move away from notions of 'location of disturbance to location of difference'.

Reem Shelhi's chapter 'How We Came To Live In Stuckness: Intersectional Axes of Oppression and "Affectivism" as a Group Analytic Intervention' is a personal inquiry that 'moves beyond an academic paper to the lived experience of the roots of intersectionality'. Shelhi's uncompromising account sees the 'group analytic setting as a microcosm of the larger cultural-socio-political environment'. In Chapter 4, Shelhi draws on Fanon's work to show 'how different axes of oppression can interlock, forming sedimented intersectional knots of stuckness and immobility that, if overlooked, ignored or denied find explosive' expression'. Shelhi coins the term 'Affectivism' to show how affectivism can 'transform locations of disturbance into locations of discovery, espousing a curious rather than curative approach'. Shelhi's personal grappling with the 'not enough problem' will speak to people in group analytic therapy, training, practice, and institutions who hold intersectional positions of identity and context that are marginalized and silenced. Shelhi proposes seven strands of her intersectional identity, which she juxtaposes with associated acts of oppression. Shelhi locates these in the liminal spaces of therapeutic group work comprising of (1) Race, Ethnicity and Culture (Psychoanalytic Supremacy), (2) Gender (Misogynoir), (3) Sexuality (Homophobia), (4) Religion (Islamophobia and Rationalisation), (5) Class (Splitting), Political Allegiances (Pinkwashing), (6) Ability ('Disorder' Pathologies), (6) Political Allegiance, and (7) Ability ('Disorder' Pathologies). Shelhi's chapter demonstrates that 'although these abstracted identity classifications are set out in a linear way, they are inextricably bound up, representing micro, macro and meso nodal points of a system larger than the sum of its parts'.

Farideh Dizadji and Suryia Nayak's chapter 'An intersectional response to the intersectionality of trauma' is in the form of a conversation that parallels the method of free-floating conversation in therapeutic groups. Their conversation draws on personal and clinical material to focus on situations and experiences of the extreme trauma of political refugees. In Chapter 5, Dizadji and Nayak argue that

> *concepts of trauma need to be continually reinvented and re-understood within the political, social, and cultural contexts in which traumatization occurs. More specifically, we argue that trauma is intersectional in its constitution and experience, and as such, the evolution of conceptual frameworks about trauma needs to be intersectional. The trauma experienced by refugees cannot be viewed simply in terms of subjective personal trauma but must be understood and worked with in terms of the political contexts that (re)produce trauma.*

Their conversation reflects on three interrelated questions:

1   Under the lens of intersectionality, what does it feel like to be traumatized, and is it possible to understand these feelings as intersectional?
2   How do we relate to the intersectionality of trauma for a person or group?
3   How can intersectionality enable an articulation of the basic aim of therapy with reference to trauma?

Alasdair Forrest's chapter, 'Diffraction as the Group-Specific Phenomenon', takes an intersectional concept from feminist science studies and applies it to the group-analytic situation. In Chapter 6, he argues that the mirror reaction is a limiting concept that makes it hard to consider the breadth of intersectional identities that are always alive in groups. He argues that Group Analysis must respond to the challenge to be conceptually open and says that the ideas that launched the group-analytic project risk rusting away if they are not re-examined. He says that intersectionality provides a truly Foulkesian way of doing this because it retains an interest in the material, bodily reality as the anchoring point while also theorizing how people are positioned by the operation of power in their lives. He proposes a change to conducting to account for racist dynamics in groups.

Dick Blackwell and Claire Bacha's chapter 'Missing Dialogues' is constructed from an excerpt from their email correspondence between September 2021–November 2021. Blackwell and Bacha's correspondence was prompted by their attendance at a group organizing a webinar to commemorate the September 2021 special issue of the journal *Group Analysis* on Racism. This is an important chapter because the correspondence between these two eminent established group analysts who have been instrumental in the development of Group Analysis holds a historical account of group analytic concepts, processes, structures, and institutional practices. The email exchange between Blackwell and Bacha in Chapter 7 grapples with the geopolitical, historical, and social contexts and processes in which Group Analysis has developed and exists. Blackwell and Bacha raise process issues that pertain to all psychotherapeutic organizations, namely how the institutional matrix of organizations is intersectional and replicates intersectional dynamics of power, privilege, and position. This is an important chapter because it shows opportunities and difficulties in applying intersectional ideas to group-analytic training and to the group-analytic corpus. Fundamentally, as it develops, the correspondents disagree on whether this constitutes a dialogue at all. Bacha suggests it does, while Blackwell feels that these points he has been making for years are not taken up, which defeats the prospect of dialogue. Both correspondents claim that the other is missing them, or that they are missing something, or being missed. Bacha and Blackwell's trope of what is absent, present, visible, and hidden is a theme threaded throughout the whole of this book. The resounding message is that the lens of intersectionality shines a light on the power dynamics that construct what is absent and present, visible and not visible. Making the hidden visible and giving a name to the nameless is the heart of psychodynamic practice. The misconception is that psychotherapeutic concepts of the 'unconscious', including projective identification, resonance, and countertransference, are enough to excavate the psychic defences against the compound injuries of being in the intersection of social inequalities. This book calls for the conceptualization of an intersectional unconscious and intersectional defences. The point is we are all intersectional beings, and as such, it makes no sense to formulate or apply therapeutic interventions and frameworks that are not intersectional.

It is hoped that the intersection of positions that form this book on intersectionality and group therapy contributes to putting intersectionality to work in a move from shying away from the words rhetorical political correctness to intersectional-orientated clinical action. The future and the relevance of Group Analysis and other modalities of psychodynamic therapy depend on a mutually constitutive exchange between intersectionality and psychoanalytic theories. The future and efficacy of Group Analysis and other modalities of psychodynamic therapy urgently need to shift to a decolonized experience, culture, and framework of practice and institutional structures. The challenge and opportunity of Group Analysis's slow open theoretical group, which welcomes concepts of liberation from theories such as anti-racist, Post-colonial, Critical Race, Black feminist, and queer theory, is the experience of how, 'in motion, in transition, in movement, we must continually build a habitation for our ideas, our thoughts, and ourself' (Seshadri-Crooks, 2000:373).

References

Aiyegbusi, A. (2021a) The White Mirror: Face to Face with Racism in Group Analysis Part 1 – Mainly Theory. *Group Analysis*. https://doi.org/10.1177/0533316421992315

Aiyegbusi, A. (2021b) The White Mirror: Face to Face with Racism in Group Analysis Part 2 – Mainly Practice. *Group Analysis*. https://doi.org/10.1177/0533316421992438

Alarcón, N. (1990) The Theoretical Subject(s) of This Bridge Called My Back and Anglo-American Feminism. In Anzaldúa, G. (ed.) *Making Face, Making Soul/Haciendo Caras: Creative and Critical Perspectives by Women of Color*. San Francisco: Aunt Lute Books, pp. 356–369.

Anthias, F. (2011) Intersections and Translocations: New Paradigms for Thinking about Cultural Diversity and Social Identities. *European Educational Research Journal*, 10(2): 204–217.

Anzaldúa, G. (2007) *Borderlands/La Frontera: The New Mestiza*, 3rd ed. San Francisco: Aunt Lute Books.

Azu-Okeke, O. (2003) Response to Lecture by Dick Blackwell. *Group Analysis*, 36(4): 465–476. https://doi.org/10.1177/0533316403364003

Bhavnani, K. (ed.) (2001) *Feminism and 'Race'*. Oxford: Oxford University Press.

Biran, H. (2014) The Intersubjective and Social Unconscious Are Inseparable. *Group Analysis*, 47(3): 283–292.

Blackwell, D. (2003) Colonialism and Globalization: A Group Analytic Perspective. 27th S.H. Foulkes Annual Lecture. *Group Analysis*, 36(4): 445–463.

Blackwell, D. (2014) Racism and the Unconscious. Review of M. Fakhry Davids, Internal Racism: A Psychoanalytic Approach to Race and Difference. *Group Analysis*, 47(3): 345–355.

Boyce Davies, C. (1994) *Black Women, Writing and Identity: Migrations of the Subject*. London: Routledge.

Boyce Davies, C. (2013) *Caribbean Spaces: Escapes from Twilight Zones*. Chicago: University of Illinois Press.

Brah, A. (1996) *Cartographies of Diaspora: Contesting Identities*. Abingdon: Routledge.

Brah, A. and Phoenix, A. (2004) Ain't IA Woman? Revisiting Intersectionality. *Journal of International Women's Studies*, 5(3): 75–87.

Brown, D. (1997) Conversation with Norbert Elias. *Group Analysis*, 30(4): 515–524.

Burman, E. and Frosh, S. (2005) Editorial Introduction: Group Analysis Special Issue New Currents in Contemporary Social Theory and Implications for Group-Analytic Theory and Practice. *Group Analysis*, 38(1): 7–15.

Butler, J. (1997) Burning Acts, Injurious Speech. In Salih, S. with Butler, J. (eds.) (2004) *The Judith Butler Reader*. Oxford: Blackwell Publishing Ltd., pp. 212–239.

Butler, J. (1999) Preface. In Butler, J. (ed.) (2006) *Gender Trouble: Feminism and the Subversion of Identity*, 3rd ed. New York: Routledge [Originally published in 1990 by Routledge].

Cade Bambara, T. (ed.) (2005) *The Black Woman: An Anthology*. New York: Washington Square Press, pp. 123–135.

Caselli, D. (2005) *Beckett's Dantes: Intertextuality in the Fiction and Criticism*. Manchester: Manchester University Press.

Chantler, K. (2005) From Disconnection to Connection: 'Race', Gender and the Politics of Therapy. *British Journal of Guidance & Counselling*, 33(2): 239–256. https://doi.org/10.1080/03069880500132813

Cho, S., Crenshaw, K. W., and McCall, L. (2013) Toward a Field of Intersectionality Studies: Theory, Applications and Praxis. *Signs: Journal of Women and Culture in Society*, 38(4): 785–810.

Christian, B. (1987) The Race for Theory. In James, J. and Sharpley-Whiting, T. D. (eds.) (2000) *The Black Feminist Reader*. Oxford: Blackwell Publishers Ltd., pp. 11–23.

The Combahee River Collective (1977) A Black Feminist Statement. In James, J. and Sharpley-Whiting, T. D. (eds.) (2000) *The Black Feminist Reader*. Oxford: Blackwell Publishers Ltd., pp. 261–270.

Cooper, A. J. (2017 [1982]) *A Voice from the South: By a Black Woman of the South*. Chapel Hill, NC: University of North Carolina Press.

Crenshaw, K. (1989) Demarginalizing the Intersection of Race and Sex: A Black Feminist Critique of Antidiscrimination Doctrine, Feminist Theory and Antiracist Politics. *The University of Chicago Legal Forum. Feminism in the Law: Theory, Practice and Criticism*, 1989: 139–167.

Crenshaw, K. (1991) Mapping the Margins: Intersectionality, Identity Politics, and Violence Against Women of Color. *Stanford Law Review*, 43(6): 1241–1299.

Crenshaw, K. (2017) *On Intersectionality: Essential Writings*. New York: The New Press.

Dalal, F. (1998) *Taking the Group Seriously: Towards a Post-Foulkesian Group Analytic Theory*. London: Jessica Kingsley Publishers.

Dalal, F. (2001) The Social Unconscious: A Post-Foulkesian Perspective. *Group Analysis*, 34(4): 539–555.

Davis, A. Y. (1971) Reflections on the Black Woman's Role in the Community of Slaves. *The Black Scholar*, 3(4): 2–15.

Davis, A. Y. (1981) *Women, Race and Class*. New York: Vintage Books.

Elias, N. (1978) *What Is Sociology?* New York: Columbia University Press.

Elias, N. (1999) Introdução à sociologia. Translation by Maria Luísa Ribeiro Ferreira. Lisboa: Edições 70. In Quintaneiro, T. (ed.) (2004) *The Concept of Figuration or Configuration in Norbert Elias' Sociological Theory. Teoria & Sociedade*, 2. http://socialsciences.scielo.org/scielo.php?pid=S1518-44712006000200002&script=sci_abstract

Fotopoulou, A. (2012) Intersectionality Queer Studies and Hybridity: Methodological Frameworks for Social Research. *Journal of International Women's Studies*, 13(2): 19–32.

Foucault, M. (1975) *The Birth of the Clinic: An Archaeology of Medical Perception*. Trans. A. M. Sheridan Smith. New York: Vintage.

Foucault, M. (1980) *Power/Knowledge: Selected Interviews and Other Writings*. Ed. C. Gordon. New York: Pantheon Press, pp. 1972–1977.

Foucault, M. (1993 [1982]) The Subject and Power. In Dreyfus, H. L. and Rabinow, P. (eds.) *Michel Foucault: Beyond Structuralism and Hermeneutics*, 2nd ed. Chicago, IL: University of Chicago Press, pp. 208–226.

Foulkes, E. (ed.) (1990) *Selected Papers of S. H. Foulkes: Psychoanalysis and Group Analysis*. London: Karnac Books.

Foulkes, S. H. (1948 [1984]) *Introduction to Group-Analytic Psychotherapy: Studies in the Social Interaction of Individuals and Groups*. London: Karnac [Original publication, London: Heinemann].

Foulkes, S. H. (1964) *Therapeutic Group Analysis*. London: Allen and Unwin [Reprinted London: Karnac, 1984].

Foulkes, S. H. (1975) *The Group-Analytic Situation in Group-Analytic Psychotherapy: Methods and Principles*. London: Karnac.

Foulkes, S. H. (1986) *Group Analytic Psychotherapy: Methods and Principles*. London: Karnac Books.

Garland, C. (2010) *The Groups Book: Psychoanalytic Group Therapy: Principles and Practice, Including the Groups Manual: A Treatment Manual with Clinical Vignettes*. London: Karnac.

Grzanka, P. R. (2014) *Intersectionality: A Foundations and Frontiers Reader*. Boulder, CO: Westview Press.

Grzanka, P. R. (2020) From Buzzword to Critical Psychology: An Invitation to Take Intersectionality Seriously. *Women & Therapy*, 43(3–4): 244–261.

Gunnarsson, L. (2017) Why We Keep Separating the 'Inseparable': Dialecticizing Intersectionality. *European Journal of Women's Studies*, 24(2): 114–127.

Hill Collins, P. (2000) *Black Feminist Thought: Knowledge, Consciousness, and the Politics of Empowerment*, 2nd ed. London: Routledge.

Hopper, E. (1982) The Problem of Context. *Group Analysis*, 15(2): 136–157.

Hopper, E. (1997) Traumatic Experience in the Unconscious Life of Groups: A Fourth Basic Assumption. *Group Analysis*, 30(4): 439–470.

Hopper, E. (2003) *The Social Unconscious: Selected Papers*. London: Jessica Kingsley Publishers.

Hopper, E. and Weinberg, H. (eds.) (2011) *The Social Unconscious in Persons, Groups, and Societies. Volume I: Mainly Theory*. London: Karnac.

Huggan, G. (1989) Decolonizing the Map. *Ariel*, 20(4): 115–131.

Hull, G. T., Bell Scott, P. and Smith, B. (eds.) (1982) *All the Women Are White, All the Blacks Are Men, But Some of Us Are Brave*. New York: The Feminist Press.

Ilmonen, K. (2019) Identity Politics Revisited: On Audre Lorde, Intersectionality, and Mobilizing Writing Styles. *European Journal of Women's Studies*, 26(1): 7–22.

Ken, I. (2008) Beyond the Intersection: A New Culinary Metaphor for Race-Class-Gender Studies. *Sociological Theory*, 26(2): 152–172.

Knauss, W. (2006) The Group in the Unconscious: A Bridge between the Individual and the Society. *Group Analysis*, 39(2): 159–170.

Lavie, L. (2005) The Lost Roots of the Theory of Group Analysis: 'Taking Interrelational Individuals Seriously'! *Group Analysis*, 38(4): 519–535.

Liveras, M. (2020) Positions and Figurations in Group Analytic Psychotherapy: An Account of Therapeutic Processes in the Individual as Part of the Group. *Group Analysis*, 53(1): 20–36. https://doi.org/10.1177/0533316419881850

Lorde, A. (1977) The Transformation of Silence into Language and Action. In Lorde, A. (ed.) (1984) *Sister Outsider: Essays and Speeches*. Trumansburg: The Crossing Press, pp. 40–44.

Lorde, A. (1984) *Sister Outsider: Essays and Speeches*. Trumansburg: The Crossing Press.

McCall, L. (2005) The Complexity of Intersectionality. *Signs: Journal of Women in Culture and Society*, 30(3): 1771–1800.

McKinnon, C. (2013) Intersectionality as Method: A Note. *Signs: Journal of Women in Culture and Society*, 38(4): 1019–1030.

Milivojevic, L. (2005) Importance of Projective Identification Influence on Countertransference in a Traumatized Group. *Group Analysis*, 38(2): 237–248.

Minh-ha, T. T. (1991) *When the Moon Waxes Red: Representation, Gender and Cultural Politics*. New York: Routledge.

Mirza, H. S. and Gunaratnam, Y. (2014) 'The Branch on Which I Sit': Reflections on Black British Feminism Author(s). *Feminist Review*, 108: 125–133.

Mohanty, C. T. (2003) *Feminism Without Borders: Decolonizing Theory, Practicing Solidarity*. Durham: Duke University Press.

Nayak, S. (2017) 'Location as Method' in Special Issue on 'Bordering, Exclusions and Necropolitics'. *Qualitative Research*, 17(3): 202–216.

Nayak, S. (2020a) Intersectionality with an Eye to Psychotherapy Clinical and Professional Ethics. In *Oxford Handbook of Psychotherapy and Ethics*. Oxford: Oxford University Press.

Nayak, S. (2020b) A Response to: 'Intimate Others and the Othering of Intimates: The Gendered Psycho-Politics of the Entangled Relational' by Farhad Dalal (Dalal, 2020)'. *Group Analysis*, 53(4): 451–462. https://doi.org/10.1177/0533316420969592

Nayak, S. (2021a) Black Feminist Intersectionality Is Vital to Group Analysis: Can Group Analysis Allow Outsider Ideas In? *Group Analysis*, 54(3): 337–353.

Nayak, S. (2021b) Racialized Misogyny: Response to 44th Foulkes Lecture. *Group Analysis*, 54(4): 520–527. https://doi.org/10.1177/05333164211039983

Nayak, S. (2022) An Intersectional Model of Reflection: Is Social Work Fit for Purpose in an Intersectionally Racist World? *Critical Radical Social Work*, 10(2).

Nitzgen, D. (2001) Training in Democracy, Democracy in Training: Notes on Group Analysis and Democracy. *Group Analysis*, 34(3): 331–347.

Phoenix, A. and Pattynama, P. (eds.) (2006) Special Issue on 'Intersectionality'. *European Journal of Women's Studies*, 13(3): 187–192.

Pichon-Rivière, E. (1979) *Teoría del vínculo* [Theory of the Bond]. Buenos Aires: Nueva Visión.

Pilgrim, D. and Rogers, A. (2008) Socioeconomic Disadvantage. In Tummey, R. and Turner, T. (eds.) *Critical Issues in Mental Health*. Basingstoke: Palgrave Macmillan, pp. 23–40.

Pines, M. (2014) The 'Isms' in Groups: Conflict and Difference. *Group Analysis*, 47(3_ suppl): 42–49.

Probyn, E. (2003) The Spatial Imperative of Subjectivity. In Anderson, K., Domosh, M., Pile, S. and Thrift, N. (eds.) *Handbook of Cultural Geography*. London: Sage Publications Ltd., pp. 290–299.

Purkayastha, B. (2012) Intersectionality in a Transnational World. *Gender and Society*, 26(1): 55–66.

Radhakrishnan, R. (2000) Postmodernism and the Rest of the World. In Afzal-Khan, F. and Seshadri-Crooks, K. (eds.) *The Pre-occupation of Postcolonial Studies*. Durham: Duke University Press, pp. 37–70.

Raufman, R. and Weinberg, H. (2016) Early Mother – Son Relationships, Primary Levels of Mental Organization and the Foundation Matrix as Expressed in Fairy Tales: The Case of the 'Jewish Mother'. *Group Analysis*, 49(2): 149–163.

Razack, S. (1998) *Looking White People in the Eye: Gender, Race, and Culture in Courtrooms and Classrooms*. Toronto: University of Toronto Press.

Rodó-Zárate, M. and Jorba, M. (2022) Metaphors of Intersectionality: Reframing the Debate with a New Proposal. *European Journal of Women's Studies*, 29(1): 23–38.

Rohr, E. (2014) 38th S.H. Foulkes Annual Lecture: Intimacy and Social Suffering in a Globalized World. *Group Analysis*, 47(4): 365–383.

Rohr, E. (2018) World in Motion – The Emotional Impact of Mass Migration. *Group Analysis*, 51(3): 283–296.

Scholz, R. (2004) Self-Esteem and the Process of Its Re-Assessment in Multicultural Groups: Renegotiating the Symbolic Social Order. *Group Analysis*, 37(4): 525–535.

Seshadri-Crooks, K. (2000) Surviving Theory: A Conversation with Homi K. Bhabha. In Afzal-Khan, F. and Seshadri-Crooks, K. (eds.) *The Pre-occupation of Postcolonial Studies*. Durham: Duke University Press, pp. 369–379.

Taylor, K.-Y. (ed.) (2017) *How We Get Free: Black Feminism and the Combahee River Collective*. Chicago: Haymarket Books.

Treacher, A. (2005) On Postcolonial Subjectivity. *Group Analysis*, 38(1): 43–57.

Truth, S. (1851) Ain't I A Woman? In Collins, O. (ed.) (1998) *Speeches That Changed the World*. Louisville: Westminster John Knox Press, pp. 208–209.

Tubert-Oklander, J. (2019) Beyond Psychoanalysis and Group Analysis. The Urgent Need for a New Paradigm of the Human Being. *Group Analysis*, 52(4): 409–426.

Tucker, S. (2011) Psychotherapy Groups for Traumatized Refugees and Asylum Seekers. *Group Analysis*, 44(1): 68–82.

Walker, A. (1982) *The Color Purple*. New York: Washington Square Press.

Weegmann, M. (2014) *The World within the Group: Developing a Theory for Group Analysis*. London: Karnac.

Weinberg, H. (2007) So What Is This Social Unconscious Anyway? *Group Analysis*, 40(3): 307–322.

Winker, G. and Degele, N. (2011) Intersectionality as Multi-Level Analysis: Dealing with Social Inequality. *European Journal of Women's Studies*, 18(1): 51–66.

Yuval-Davis, N. (2014) Intersectionality, Inequality and Bordering Processes. *Presented at the Conference: XVIII ISA World Congress of Sociology*, Yokohama, Japan.

Chapter 1

Holding the Broken Pieces

An Intersectional Approach to Group Analysis for Women in Prison

Anne Aiyegbusi

Introduction

The focus of this chapter is on integrating principles of intersectionality to strengthen and enhance group analytic therapy for incarcerated women with complex emotional needs as reflected in their histories of trauma, abuse and offending and in their being psychiatrically diagnosed with personality disorders. Intersectionality is felt to be particularly relevant for this work because it is:

- A framework offering the analytic capacity to understand the impact of multiple marginalised identities
- Rooted in the lived experience of socially and politically oppressed and voiceless persons
- Committed to holding together and integrating all the parts of a person or community that has become fragmented with many labels, borders and divisions

Women who are convicted of offences are typically stigmatised to the point of being excluded from definitions of womanhood. Incarcerated women are grouped together, excluded in ill-fitting, closed institutions and frequently denigrated. As such, it can be tempting to offer blanket and concrete responses to what are complex stories and needs. The pressure to try to convert complexity into simplicity may feel overwhelming, mirroring the women's internal struggles with uncontainable and typically unfathomable emotional experiences, which are also implicated in their offending. Such strategies may offer short-term illusionary solutions that later fall apart as the unprocessed phenomena of trauma once again spill out and overwhelm.

In this chapter, consideration will be given to how group therapy enhanced by the particular anti-discriminatory rigour provided by intersectionality might offer an effective therapeutic approach for convicted and incarcerated women prisoners diagnosed with personality disorders. Like many incarcerated women, those who are members of the group represented in this chapter have complex histories of attachment trauma and/or interpersonal abuse with convictions for offending against others, including violently. All are vulnerable to marginalisation and

DOI: 10.4324/9781003232216-2

exclusion across multiple axes of identity. As will be seen through a representative clinical example, this approach may help women find, despite their differences, common ground, enabling them to come together in mutual solidarity and support to address the suffering and exclusion that unites them.

The Complex Needs of Incarcerated Women

Women who come into contact with the criminal justice system through offending, including those whose ultimate detention is in prison or secure mental health settings, are among society's most disadvantaged and vulnerable persons. Women sentenced to imprisonment who are also diagnosed with personality disorders by definition have a number of interlocking identities, which together render them vulnerable to oppression and erasure. That is, their gender, the fact of their being imprisoned offenders and sufferers of mental health problems, including the controversial and contested diagnosis of personality disorder (Scanlon and Adlam, 2022). This canopy of constructs conceals a multiplex of other complex, devastating and what are often personally felt to be broken parts beyond individual women's capacity to hold together. Within the criminal justice system, especially the carceral estate, the meaning of women's offending and any comprehensive understanding of their needs have historically been occluded within a landscape dominated by perceived male needs. They have been described as erased and subordinated in the context of male offending requirements. Indeed, it is often said that women have been force-fitted into a system designed for men (Motz et al., 2020).

Baroness Corston's (2007) review of vulnerable women in prisons concluded that women with histories of abuse are disproportionately to be found housed in these institutions, which are likely to compound the harm to which they have already been subjected. Alternative forms of response have been recommended but are yet to materialise. The late Chris Tchaikovsky, former imprisoned woman and founder of a charity for women affected by the criminal justice system entitled 'Women in Prison' is quoted in the document 'Still Dying on the Inside' by Inquest (2017:12):

> *Taking the most hurt people out of society and punishing them in order to teach them how to live within society is at best, futile. Whatever else a prisoner knows, she knows everything there is to know about punishment because that is exactly what she has grown up with. Whether it is childhood sexual abuse, indifference, neglect; punishment is most familiar to her.*

Within the women's prison population, Black and other minority ethnic women fare worst of all. In the foreword to the Prison Reform Trust and Hibiscus Initiatives (2017:2) publication entitled 'Counted Out: Black, Asian and Minority Ethnic Women in the Criminal Justice System', Larasi comments on the injustices and inequalities that are rife within the system, impacting Black and Asian prisoners and says: 'We also know that women and girls routinely face multiple, intersecting inequalities and that the criminal justice system is too often the "hard face" of this injustice'. Black women in prison constitute a population who experience myriad disadvantages, inequalities and other burdens to a disproportionate degree. For example, they are over-represented in prison populations and receive harsher sentences. Black women in prison are more likely to head single-parent households, are more likely to be foreign nationals, experience language barriers in prison, to have suffered female genital mutilation and to have been trafficked and involved in prostitution. With regard to mental health difficulties, Black women are less likely to receive support for their distress, which in turn is more likely to be conceptualised in terms of anger management problems. They are more likely to be subject to segregation. Friendships and interactions with other Black women are likely to be subject to suspicion and regarded as gang activity. The absence of contact with Black women who are in a position of influence compounds their disadvantaged and oppressed positioning. In terms of day-to-day contact in prison, there is an under-representation of Black staff who are also subject to surveillance and suspicion (Inquest, 2017; Prison Reform Trust and Hibiscus Initiatives, 2017). Aiyegbusi (2020) analysed the tragic experience of Sarah Reed, who killed herself in 2016 while remanded to Holloway prison and was suffering acute psychological distress. Aiyegbusi (2020) demonstrated how forensic mental health and criminal justice institutions are capable of reproducing extreme racial trauma more typical of bygone centuries for Black women who, like Sarah Reed, are rendered particularly vulnerable by virtue of their personal experiences of abuse at the intersection of race and gender, traumatic loss and consequent mental health distress.

Group Analysis and Foulkes's Matrix

This section considers a core element of group analysis, Foulkes's construction of a matrix.

S.H. Foulkes described a collection of group analytic constructs and specific factors which function to operationalise the group as a therapeutic modality. Of them all, the abstraction he called the matrix has been described as the most fundamental. Nitzgen and Hopper (2017:15) describe the matrix as 'the cornerstone of the theory of group analysis'. Foulkes and Anthony (1957) initially thought of the matrix as a form of neural network with individual group members perceived in terms of nodal points through which all communications and experiences pass. Foulkes (1975) perceived the matrix as the theatre of operations for all mental processes in the group. This was analogous to the human mind being the theatre of operations for all mental processes in an individual person. With regard to the group matrix, Foulkes conceptualised group processes, piercing right through and effectively impaling individuals who take up and verbalise specific concerns. Those concerns affect the whole group but may be personified by an individual protagonist whose valency (Bion, 1961) renders them the best candidate within that group for becoming the location of disturbance, of which the scapegoat may be considered an exemplar. In such circumstances, a core task of the group is for individual members to recognise and integrate the parts of themselves located within the disturbance currently carried by a sole member.

Foulkes's work on the matrix has been widely considered incomplete (Dalal, 1998; Roberts, 1982), with other group analytic authors and researchers taking his seminal theories forward. Building on Foulkes's work, which eventually included a somewhat embryonic further concept of a personal matrix, Nitzgen and Hopper (2017) conceptualised the entire group matrix as a 'tripartite structure'. Thus, today the matrix is generally recognised as comprising three overlapping and interpenetrating matrices in the form of the personal matrix, the dynamic matrix and the foundation matrix. As Nitzgen and Hopper (2017:16) state:

> personal *matrices of the group members all feed into (and are modified by) the* dynamic *matrix of the group. Simultaneously and recursively the foundation matrix is activated, and, in turn, feeds into the dynamic matrix in a recursive, circular loop. . . . The group matrix as a whole links time and space in such a way that the past can be presented in the present, and the present can be manifest simultaneously in several spaces.*

The personal matrix is posited as reflecting the individualised experiences and personality composition of members based upon their specific make-up, background and lives lived (Nitzgen and Hopper, 2017). The dynamic matrix is regarded as emerging through the relationships and interactions that take place once the group has developed. The dynamic matrix continues to develop in an iterative way throughout the life of the group. From the perspective of the group analytic model, the foundation matrix is a relatively static part of the overall matrix, which consists of what group members bring to the group that is shared. Even if they are total strangers, members are regarded as being of the same species with the same cultural and biological heritage. Shared cultural heritage includes being bound together by a shared worldview about how life is lived, including basic rituals of daily living, such as the use of language (Pines, 2000). Foulkes (1990) viewed the way in which people can become bound together by unconscious forces as evidence of a shared foundation matrix. However, the commonality of experience brought by group members to the foundation matrix has been contested. A more or less uniform idea of a foundation matrix may not help to represent disturbance that results from difference.

Intersectionality

Intersectionality offers a perspective rooted in the experiences of those whose voices have been excluded from mainstream narratives. At root, it is an analytic tool for giving voice to the lived experiences of multi-axes discriminations encountered by Black women. Recognised as a Black feminist ideology, intersectionality provides a critical perspective of dominant understandings of race, gender, sexuality, class and other socially constructed, hierarchised dimensions of human identity. The experience of those typically considered 'other' are placed central, taking account of how the dominant, frequently middle-class, male, heterosexual, white supremacist discourse impacts life chances. From mental health and criminal justice perspectives, intersectional theory would recognise the role of social experience, especially how structural inequalities, marginalisation and discrimination function as vehicles for transporting social pathology to its location with particular, vulnerable people, populations and identities.

Although subject to some controversy as to what she actually said, Sojourner Truth's (1851) speech entitled 'Women's Rights' delivered at a Convention held in Akron, Ohio, has been characterised as a plea for inclusion. The plea was: 'Ain't I a Woman?' Truth's speech is credited as the first recorded intersectional narrative. It highlighted the intersection of race and gender by challenging the way that Black men and white women both erased the details of lives, traumas and often insurmountable social obstacles blocking equity for Black women. Kimberlé Crenshaw (1989) coined the actual term intersectionality. She did so in a legal context whereby she proposed it as an analytical framework for capturing and elaborating on the precise nature of discrimination that occurs when there are multiple axes of identity vulnerable to oppression. The people Crenshaw represented were typically Black, working-class women who had previously been erased and subsumed within the normative and more power-advantaged accounts of single-axis discrimination that were experienced by white women and Black men. These accounts failed to represent Black women who were allocated ever closer to the margins, experienced worse discrimination than either white women or Black men, and who, because of accepted standards, were unable to demonstrate this and, therefore, defend their claims. There was no recognised framework to capture the discrimination they faced prior to Crenshaw's intersectional framework.

Importantly, intersectional frameworks emphasise the way that the whole tends to be greater than the sum of its parts when considering the burden of multiple interlocking identities vulnerable to oppression and exclusion. As an analytic framework, intersectionality therefore also offers a way to recognise patterns of conscious and unconscious discriminatory processes, such as the dynamics maintaining hierarchical structures of power, privilege and position. This includes communities of advantage and disadvantage perpetuating insider/outsider statuses. Particular tropes and stereotypes typically emerge through projective processes whereby those in power rid themselves of unwanted characteristics by locating them in the vulnerable and marginalised, thus further assuring their positional power and sense of superiority. The empirical knowledge underpinning intersectionality is drawn from lived experiences of oppression, developed and shaped over centuries of denied reality and, therefore, typically 'underground' networks and communities of otherwise voiceless peoples. Although its foundations are firmly in Black feminism and critical race theory, since Crenshaw's (1989) seminal work, intersectionality has been used as an analytic and organising framework for a vast range of political, social and clinical contexts where complex and multi-axial discrimination is at its core (for example, Friedman et al., 2020; Hamad, 2019; Hill Collins and Bilge, 2016; Kinouani, 2021; Potter, 2015; Turner, 2021).

Finding that traditional Foulkesian group analysis fails to reflect or meet the needs of diverse populations within the UK, especially where there are interlocking and multi-axial identities vulnerable to erasure and/or oppression, a number of Group Analytic authors of colour have introduced intersectional thinking into their writings (Aiyegbusi, 2021a, 2021b; Kent, 2021; Nayak, 2020, 2021; Stevenson, 2020). These authors argue that traditional group analytic theories and practices recreate oppressive, harmful and traumatising, hierarchal and excluding cultures. They recommend the integration of intersectional frameworks to mitigate the consequent risks to the health and wellbeing of minority members from underrepresented and concomitantly misrepresented populations and to level the playing field in terms of potentially equitable treatment outcomes. In light of these recommendations, the usefulness of an intersectional approach to group analysis for convicted and incarcerated women with complex presentations, including multi-axial identities of stigma and oppression, is explored in this chapter.

Intersectional Matrix

The term intersectional matrix is used here to capture the interaction of multiple facets of identity and the way these emerge and play out within the matrix of an analytic group. In the context of the tripartite system, the matrix will be considered in terms of personal, dynamic and foundation matrices. Key to establishing the value of integrating an intersectional approach is whether the matrix is able to hold and contain the multiplicity of interlocking identities brought to it by the women's personal intersectional matrices. This is especially relevant to the enormity of intertwined, mutually reinforcing traumatogenic and criminogenic phenomena involved. Can this be held and contained sufficiently to offer the promise of future integration, first for the group and then by internalisation for individual members? Can this approach help the women to, in Nayak's (2021:339) words, 'grapple with the excruciating difficulty of lying down with the interconnected parts' of themselves as a group and as individuals?

The intersectional matrix (Table 1.1) represents group members' personal matrices, which were brought to the foundation matrix of the group. Can these complex dimensions of identity possibly be held in order to find a way to lie down together and be held within a co-created dynamic matrix? Might the emergent tripartite intersectional matrix then function as a secure base providing what Stein (2022:172) describes as 'integration of emotional narrative and affective states'?

Intersectional, Tripartite Structure

As can be seen, despite essentially being a homogenous group for convicted and imprisoned women offenders diagnosed with personality disorders, the personal matrices of the group members are diverse in terms of the range of other axes of identity represented. This includes immediate and ancestral nationality, age, religion, race, culture, ethnicity, gender and sexual identity, class, physical health and

Table 1.1 Women's Group – Intersectional Matrix

Name	Age	Siblings	Sexual Orientation	Ethnic Background	Health and Ableness	Developmental Information	Education and Employment	Relationships	Offending
Amina	36	Only child	Hetero-sexual	Black African of Muslim faith. Born in Somalia.	Dyslexia. Suffered female genital mutilation. Currently has psychiatric diagnoses of antisocial and emotionally unstable personality disorders with PTSD. Has history of addictions.	Fled civil war as a refugee with parents during early childhood. Lived in detention centres, hostels and social housing, frequently in poverty. Witnessed domestic violence. Father had alcohol problems. Mother had mental health problems and was hospitalised on occasion. Sexual exploitation and physical abuse in drug gangs.	Struggled academically due to trauma and dyslexia. Groomed and drawn into drug gangs in teens. Pimped by boyfriend.	While subject to sexual exploitation in drugs gang, gave birth to twins at age 19. Twins taken into care and adopted. Later, in relationship with violent gang member, there was domestic violence.	History of drugs-related offending after twins were adopted. Short custodial sentences. Index offence occurred while engaged in prostitution, when in a rage, she knifed a violent client who tried to rape her. Convicted of manslaughter on the grounds of diminished responsibility.
Fleur	59	Middle of three sisters	Lesbian	White, UK and secular Jewish.	Born with curvature of the spine. Hospitalised for a considerable period of time as a child due to this. Left with pronounced back deformity. Has psychiatric diagnoses of	Middle class, privileged background. Parents were successful but often absent emotionally and physically. Different from sisters, regarded as remote, introverted and uspends.	Privately uspend. Successful academically but bullied throughout schooling. Attended university. Afterwards, worked as a university research uspends.	Regarded as an asexual loner. Developed an obsessive relationship with a female lecturer whom she stalked while at university. After death of her mother,	Received a caution and agreed to have counselling following stalking of female lecturer. Convicted of kidnapping and assault for attacking female colleague/stalking victim's partner.

| | | | | | Schizoid and obsessional compulsive personality disorders. | Thought to be related to hospitalisation and physical health condition, which led to bullying by other children. | | she again uspends an obsessive relationship with a female colleague whom she stalked. This led to index offence. | Received two years uspends sentence, which she breached. |
| Jodie | 24 | Only child | Hetero-sexual | White, UK and Christian, Protestant faith. | Has self-harmed since age ten. Received treatment for addictions and trauma. Has psychiatric diagnosis of antisocial personality disorder and complex PTSD. | Taken into care as a baby due to severe neglect and abuse. Little contact with biological family and subject to over 20 foster placements. Considered 'too disturbed and destructive' and eventually remained in long term local authority care. Groomed and trafficked by paedophiles who subjected her to extreme sexual and physical violence. Believed herself to be the girlfriend of one married gang member 30 years her senior. | Did not complete compulsory education. Groomed, trafficked and sexually exploited in childhood. No adult employment | Deeply invested in paedophile gang where she had been groomed and believed herself to be the girlfriend of a married gang member 30 years her senior. Protected gang and refused to testify against them. | History of violence related to protection and loss of paedophile abuser. Index offence occurred shortly after being placed in isolated council flat as care leaver. Held up a taxi driver at knifepoint and robbed him. Convicted of armed robbery. |

(Continued)

Table 1.1 (Continued)

Name	Age	Siblings	Sexual Orientation	Ethnic Background	Health and Ableness	Developmental Information	Education and Employment	Relationships	Offending
						When grooming, gang was convicted. She assaulted a number of people and was transferred to secure care until 18 years old.			
Ella	35	Youngest of three sisters	Heterosexual	White, UK and Christian, Protestant faith.	Has psychiatric diagnoses of depression and dissociative disorder. Has a history of post-partum depression and Fabricated or Induced Illness.	Born into stable, lower middle-class family. Mother experienced post-partum depression at the time of her birth. Treated in mother and baby unit. Mother recovered but bonding remained impaired.	Attended university and qualified as a paediatric nurse.	Considered somewhat withdrawn with marked compulsive caretaking. Married in her late 20s. Had one child. Marriage broke down while she was receiving treatment for post-partum depression.	No prior history of offending or criminal conduct. Index offence occurred when her marriage broke down, and Ella began inducing illness in her child by salt overdose. The child died of renal failure and Ella was convicted of manslaughter on the grounds of diminished responsibility.

| Janis | 50 | Youngest of two children, having an older brother | Heterosexual. Since imprisonment has been able to talk about lifelong gender dysphoria. | Black, UK-born Christian, Protestant faith. Parents immigrated from Caribbean in the 1960s. | Has mild learning difficulty. Has significant scarring to body due to skin bleaching. She has no formal psychiatric diagnosis. | Born into stable and solidly working-class family. Father worked in transport department and mother was a health care assistant. Brother is now a medical doctor. Was sexually assaulted as a child and suffered racial abuse throughout school. Having a darker complexion, she was a victim of shadism by Black peers which led her to skin bleaching. | Struggled at school due to mild learning disability. Completed compulsory education with no qualifications. Always employed, working hard, sometimes holding down three jobs at once to support her family. | Long term relationship with white male partner with whom she has two children and three grandchildren. Janis was a victim of domestic violence throughout the relationship. This included physical, racial and sexual violence. He liked to re-enact master/slave sexual scenarios. Janis poisoned him to stop the abuse. She has had no contact with her children or grandchildren since arrest. | No prior offending history or criminal conduct. She was charged with poisoning her abusive partner. Janis did not defend herself by citing the prolonged domestic abuse as mitigation. She was convicted of attempted murder. |

(Continued)

Table 1.1 (Continued)

Name	Age	Siblings	Sexual Orientation	Ethnic Background	Health and Ableness	Developmental Information	Education and Employment	Relationships	Offending
Roxanne	43	Only child	Bisexual	Dual heritage, Christian, Catholic faith. Mother a white English woman. Father's heritage unknown other than he was Black.	Had mental health breakdown when mother died and received psychiatric diagnoses of emotionally unstable personality disorder and complex PTSD, which she still has. In prison, she self-harms by cutting and tying ligatures round her neck. She is also suicidal with pronounced mood instability.	Transgenerational trauma, dysfunction, care system, sexual abuse by paedophiles and chaos on mother's side of family. Mother's family also physically and racially abused Roxanne. She herself was received into local authority care on numerous occasions. Sometimes authorities activated care applications. On other occasions, she volunteered to go into care for protection from family chaos and danger. She was sexually abused by a residential care worker during one period in care.	Roxanne did well educationally. She completed an English degree and went on to train and work as a teacher with primary school children.	Has struggled to maintain relationships throughout her life and is largely solitary. She did, however, enjoy positive relationships at work with both colleagues and children.	No prior offending history or criminal conduct. The index offence occurred after Roxanne's mental health deteriorated following her mother's death. She was admitted to a mental health unit. Whilst there, she set fire to a bed. Another patient in a vulnerable state of health died of smoke inhalation. Roxanne was convicted of arson and manslaughter on the grounds of diminished responsibility.

| Sharonjit | 29 | Third of four children. Older brother and sister, younger brother. | Hetero-sexual | UK-born, of Indian heritage. Sikh faith. Grandparents on both sides of her family immigrated to UK from India. Both parents born in UK. | Had termination of pregnancy at age 13 following sexual abuse by older cousin. Suffered depression, bulimia and anorexia in university. After taking an overdose in a suicide attempt, she was admitted to a mental health unit. She currently has diagnoses of emotionally unstable personality disorder, depression and eating disorders. | Born into middle-class family. Parents and many extended family members in medical professions. Sexually abused by older male cousin for several years of childhood. Pregnancy and subsequent termination was known by large extended family, some of whom blamed her, creating significant tension. Subjected to racial abuse and bullying in school, along with taunts about the details of her abuse, pregnancy and termination. | Commenced medical school but dropped out when mental health deteriorated and she was admitted to a mental health unit. She went on to study and work in accounting, where her index offence occurred. | She has strong relationships with her immediate family members, who have supported her throughout, from pregnancy, termination, mental health problems and offending. Despite this, Sharonjit feels harshly judged by them and by people in general, which underlies her struggle to develop relationships of any kind with people. | No prior offending or history of criminal conduct. However, was found to have embezzled hundreds of thousands of pounds from the company she worked for as an accountant. She was convicted of fraud and sentenced to four years imprisonment. |

ability, family structures, educational and professional achievements, personal and generational, structural and interpersonal traumatogenic and criminogenic factors. These can be expected to influence the relational energy and dynamics within the different interrelated domains of the matrix. In particular, by producing enactments and re-enactments of conflict associated with the social implications of different combinations of identities. For example, Aiyegbusi (2021a) has described how racist enactments occur within the dynamic matrix, representing victim and perpetrator positions members and/or their ancestors have occupied in racial conflict within the social world and which have been brought to the foundation matrix, leaking into the dynamic matrix in the form of racist scenes at times of group stress and anxiety.

Stevenson (2020), in writing from the perspective of intersectional group analysis, comments on the positionality of the conductor, given that othering dynamics are inevitable when group members have suffered from structural oppression. Stevenson (2020:498) states:

I argue that a failure on behalf of the group analyst to reflexively position themselves in relation to powerful phenomena such as racism, sexism and homophobia and occurrences in the social unconscious risks a retraumatizing dynamic being paralleled in the group matrix to the detriment of group members from marginalized communities.

Kinouani (2020:64), in critically examining how whiteness organises within the tripartite group matrices, states that:

Whiteness is reproduced at all levels of human functioning. Consequently it is inevitable that it will become reproduced within the group matrix.

Kent (2021) analyses racism within a group through the prism of intersectionality, examining the phenomenon of scapegoating women of colour within analytic groups. She questions whether women of colour can ever develop through establishing intimacy with white women in analytic groups, stating:

The wounds created by oppression, whether buried deep amid historical and ancestral trauma or openly bleeding with the rawness of re-traumatization, may leave indelible stains upon our matrices.

(p. 364)

Aiyegbusi (2021b) explores an intersectional racist-sexist enactment by a subgroup, including the conductor in relation to the only Black woman in an analytic group, concluding:

This exposes the polarized expectations of black women. If not amenable to propriety as 'good', jolly, smiling help, then punished with conceptualizations of 'bad', surly, aggressive Sapphires or 'angry, black, women.

(p. 430)

Nayak (2021) asks whether group analysis can allow the anti-border ideology of intersectionality to develop its theories and practices. Emphasising the value of intersectionality to contain and hold together the otherwise potentially fragmenting or compartmentalising complexity of multi-issue oppression from structural and interpersonal trauma, Nayak (2021:342) states:

> *it seems to me that we need help to process internalized abuses or power, privilege and position, we need a decolonized framework to sharpen the political potential of group analysis.*

From the perspective of a prison therapeutic community, Parker (2007) describes how offence paralleling occurs in therapeutic groups with offenders.

Therapists

Dr Adebanjo is 53 years old. A Black UK-born woman who is a psychiatrist and group analyst, she grew up in a stable, middle-class family, the second of four children. Her three siblings are also successful professionals. Her parents immigrated to the UK from Nigeria before she was born. Dr Adebanjo is married to a man of Nigerian heritage and is the mother of two children.

Mr James is 38 years old. He is a white man and is a member of prison disciplinary staff. He works as a group facilitator on the treatment unit while training as a psychotherapist. He was born into a working-class community, the eldest of three sons. He is gay, married to a white man and they are in the process of adopting a child.

Therapists' Intersectional Preparation

As part of their commitment to integrating an intersectional approach to group therapy, the therapists engaged in thorough preparation, considering together their personal intersectional matrices and how they might emerge in the group. Each reflected on their individual location with regard to power, privilege and position across multiple dimensions of identity and how they interacted with each other. For example, as a white man, Mr James enjoys a position of considerable power and social advantage that Dr Adebanjo, as a Black woman, does not. However, Dr Adebanjo is heterosexual and a middle-class doctor. As such, she does not live with the burden of homophobia which Mr James, as a gay man, does, nor has she ever experienced the kind of financial struggle Mr James has. Then again, Mr James has not suffered generational racial trauma due to colonisation, nor does he face daily discrimination and regular hostility on the sight of his skin colour, which is compounded by gender, including how Dr Adebanjo is regularly perceived to occupy a much lower professional position than she does. As a result of their preparation, Dr Adebanjo and Mr James were able to respect each other's personal intersectional matrices and were able to learn about the multidimensional ways their intersecting axes of identity manifest in the social world and consider the probable interactions with others' intersectional matrices within a group context. From this position of knowledge and experiential learning, they were able to carefully review the personal intersectional matrices of the women who had been assessed and selected for the therapy group, hypothesising how each might inter-relate within the group based on their intersecting identities in service of co-creating the dynamic matrix.

Phases of Group Process

Three phases of the group will be described through clinical vignettes.

1   Establishing a secure base
2   What brings the house down?
3   Getting to the underbelly

First Phase – Establishing a Secure Base

The women presented and experienced themselves very much as individuals lost to the remnants of their particular lives and bruised by the carceral process so far. However, they didn't feel connected to the circumstances that had led them to imprisonment. As individuals, the overarching sense was of anxiety about each other, the therapists and themselves and what they would all encounter together. The group felt like a pool of individually wounded beings, fearful that connection might bring with it a scald. Attendance was good, mainly because the alternative was to be alone in a cell with the puzzlement and pain of their predicaments. The group eventually found common ground in the scapegoating of Ella, whose dissociated and plastered but emotionally empty smile and immaculately groomed appearance caught the attention of the other women in a negative way. This had been predicted by the therapists who were ready for the ensuing enactment. When the issue of her index offence of killing her child was raised, it was done so as a pointed accusation with sharp, alienating exclusion as the rest of the group, like a gang, turned on her. Apparently undefended, Ella came to embody, for the group, the feared scalding brought about by the exposure of offender parts of the self which had previously been protected behind personal defences. Dr Adebanjo intervened strongly at this, making it clear that the group was here to do something differently this time. They were not there to replay the past. That is, predating on the vulnerable. The women forcefully denied that a) they had preyed on vulnerable people and b) that Ella was vulnerable. In fact, the consensus was that Ella was the one who had preyed on the vulnerable; she had killed her defenceless child. Mr James said that perhaps this group could offer a place where finally they could grieve for the defenceless children the group members had been when they were harmed. It took the group a number of sessions to shift from scapegoating and brutalising strategies. Dr Adebanjo and Mr James kept the women on track, weathering the onslaught of threats to leave, favouritism accusations, accusations of being perverts themselves, of being useless, incompetent, not knowing what they are doing or not living in the real world.

Finally, the person to speak about the pain she lived with was Fleur. Perhaps unconsciously put forward by the group to try this new method, Fleur spoke quietly, a squeaking, creaking voice as though trying to push air through a vessel that had rusted through lack of use. She described the years of her childhood spent in hospital undergoing one painful surgery or procedure after another, only to eventually be allowed to go to school with other children. This glorious milestone quickly turned into a nightmare as she was bullied and pushed around. Children liked to hammer on the curvature, calling her a snail or a turtle, saying that she carried a shell on her back. The physical pain of this was excruciating, but the worst thing, she said, was that her sisters left her to endure this hideous treatment alone, ashamed to be associated with her. Resonating, Janis spoke about her own isolation at the mercy of school bullies, of being called monkey and chanted at throughout her school years and of being treated as unclean because of the colour of her skin. Other black girls, who should have been her sisters, bullied her the worst of all. Dr Adebanjo asked what kind of sisters were in this group.

After a period of silence following Dr Adebanjo's question, Roxanne said she wondered what it would be like to have people looking out for her, wanting the best for her. She couldn't imagine! The group spent a number of sessions playing with ideas about what a space would be like that worked for them as opposed to against them. Could they be the sisters they wished they'd had when most vulnerable? They realised they needed some strong ingredients such as mercy, courage, kindness, honesty, respectfulness, proper listening, sharing the space and tolerance of differences even when they didn't understand them. They agreed that these would be the rules of their 'house'. Once the women felt confident that these rules of the house could be there to stay if they worked at it, they began to talk about what had happened to them as vulnerable children and, in doing so, came to realise how they still bore the wounds and scars of this. Importantly, woman after woman realised they were no longer alone with their hellish stories. Little by little, the group began to understand that having such childhood pain in common might perhaps explain how their lives went so badly off course later on. This phase lays the ground for the work to come.

Phase Two – What Brings the House Down?

In the second phase of the group, criminogenic trauma from the foundation matrix emerged in the dynamic matrix in the form of destructiveness and enactments which broke through the stable, co-created and somewhat idealised space and rules of the house. Of all the women, Jodie was the liveliest and most inclined to test boundaries and the group culture in an upfront, sometimes aggressive way. Jodie had for some time tended to engage with Mr James in a flirtatious manner. This graduated to an increasingly sexualised narrative and enactments in the group where she regularly asked Mr James about his sexual life, suggesting it must be difficult to control himself amongst all the 'girls' he meets at work, alluding to his choosing this line of work for access to 'girls'. Mr James regularly reminded the women that his role in the group was to think with them, to help them find better and happier ways of living their lives. After a session where Jodie's questioning had been particularly penetrating, sexualised and intrusive, Mr James spoke in supervision about how anxious and threatened he was beginning to feel about her. At a deep level, he experienced Jodie as menacing. This countertransference reaction revealed clues as to what was being re-enacted within these exchanges whilst both highlighting and testing the intersections of gender difference, in particular.

In the next session, it was Amina who intervened, asking whether Jodie was confused about the relationship she has with Mr James. Roxanne asked whether it had to do with a man paying an interest in her because she herself couldn't stop wondering when Mr James's true motives would be revealed. She said a part of her trusts Mr James as a professional, and she hasn't seen him do anything to suggest otherwise, but there is a nagging part of her mind that expects his mask to slip and his true colours to be shown. Dr Adebanjo asks whether the group might consider whether it had recruited Jodie to bring out Mr James's 'true colours' so that the group would then know where it stands and where the therapist corruption lies. This question led to the women talking about the betrayals they had experienced with people who had been trusted to care for them. When Jodie was adamant that what she did was by choice, the group, led by Amina, emphasised the need to apply one of their 'rules of the house'. That is, mercy. They felt Jodie needed mercy on herself to recognise that she had deserved to be cared for, kept safe and loved as a child, ready for when she herself was an adult who could consent and be able to choose somebody for herself, not to be preyed upon by organised criminals. The group saw her as being a highly vulnerable child when she was groomed, gaslighted and exploited sexually. The group was able to think about the different ways in which abuse and lack of enough early care contributed to the way their lives had been destroyed.

Differences between those who had been fortunate to be born into stable homes, parents and families and those who had been born into chaos, abandonment and the social care system were explored, including what protection the more privileged beginnings offered and what they didn't. This led the way to exploring other differences, with tension arising around the idea of white racial privilege and thought given to how this might be lost and gained and even lost again due to vulnerability, poverty and lack of protection. But, for the women of colour, racism in their lives was constant. Amina and Janis spoke about how Dr Adebanjo, being one of the therapists for this group, made a difference to them, helping them to feel safer in the group and that they could speak about their experiences to someone who understands. And that it meant a lot to have a Black woman, a doctor, to help them feel they, too, could achieve more in life. It wasn't the usual message that they were consigned to the rubbish dump because of their race. When there were discussions about why white women couldn't have the same, Roxanne said she had been around white women in power all her life and the prison management was made up entirely of white women and white men, but she had never seen a woman of colour in any senior role which made it all the more important to have Dr Adebanjo co-facilitate the group. Sharonjit said she found it important that Dr Adebanjo and Mr James were able to work together in a caring way for the group, modelling something important, helping the women work together and feel that they could make something good out of the group. The group began to say how appreciative they were of this and compared themselves to 'a blended family' and at much the same time began to wonder whether their lives actually were fully destroyed or was there a chance of salvaging something worth living after all.

Phase 3 – Getting to the Underbelly

After the group had been running for two years, the women began to ponder what they took to calling 'the last leg'. This was a reference to looking in greater depth at the circumstances that made them different from other victimised women. What had turned them into women who hurt other people? Roxanne said they were 'hurt people who hurt people'. As was often the case when the group began to explore extremely painful matters, the first person to talk in-depth was the group member who was best placed to test the waters. On this occasion, it was Sharonjit, the woman whose offence did not include manslaughter or other forms of interpersonal violence. Sharonjit spoke about her struggle to feel complete, of always feeling there was a void and also a restless agitation and low mood she could not shake off, which exhausted her. She had discovered that stealing excited her, gave her something to look forward to and she had convinced herself she was righting a wrong due to how she felt after she had stolen. She felt complete, and the low mood, emptiness and agitation left her. But not for long, so she felt compelled to steal and steal again.

Roxanne spoke about the time she was hospitalised after the death of her mother. She had often tried to talk about her relationship with her mother, and the group was aware that it had been difficult and complicated. When her mother died, Roxanne described feeling every part of herself crash and collapse into nothing but feelings that were intolerable to bear and impossible for her to talk about. She said she wasn't thinking, just feeling, then one day, the feelings left her as if they had a life of their own. The burning feelings that had been inside her were now outside in the form of the fire she set. She set fire to a bed which for her was the bed she was born into and the bed she was raped in. When it was burning, she felt freedom. Nothing else except the mesmerising, burning bed intertwined with her feelings of freedom existed for her at the time. She had, she said, been incapable of comprehending the risk to other people.

Janis said she had poisoned her partner while he was in bed, giving him hot chocolate laced with rat poison. She had felt all those things went together. He was a rat, and he was in the bed where he had hurt and degraded her so many times for so long. And he was drinking poisoned chocolate, which she somehow felt was apt given his racist abuse, debasing and fetishising her skin colour. However, she doesn't recognise herself as that woman now. A woman so filled with hatred and anger, and so trapped that the only way she saw out of it was to poison somebody. She also had not been able to think about risks. She had lost her children and grandchildren because of what she did to her partner. And yet she is still seething inside that he hurt her so much for so long and has lost nothing, really.

Over a period of months, each woman told the story of their offence, linking it to the trauma they'd experienced and the resulting state of their mental health, which included overwhelming rage and grief, neither of which they were equipped to process and safely express due to earlier deprivations or trauma. Instead, powerful and painful feelings found expression through destructive actions. This typically occurred during periods of dissociation when devastating feelings could no longer be held in the psyche. A thread through the women's stories was that in committing their offences they had destroyed themselves. Some felt they had killed themselves and were now in a land of the living dead, and perhaps that's as good as it could ever get. Sticking steadfastly to the rules of the house, women said they felt able to get to the depth of their pain and loss, saying, thinking and sharing what they had once thought impossible. The last woman to share in depth was Ella. By the time she did, other women could offer her compassion. Their own capacity for destruction and criminality was more psychologically integrated with their woundedness, and there was less need to use Ella as the scapegoat for this. They were able to hear what Ella had lost as well as what she had stolen in the form of her child's life. Her sense of desolation and abandonment when her marriage broke down and how this reverberated with her sense of abandonment as a baby due to her mother's illness could be heard. Ella herself was less dissociated by this time, having benefitted from the group by witnessing and supporting other women as they struggled to tell their stories and understand themselves. Importantly, the holding provided by the group enabled Ella to 'go there' as the group called getting to 'the underbelly' to talk about how, in her desolation, she lost sight of her baby. She was in so much pain she didn't experience her baby as separate from her but more of a part of herself that she could use to get help in a form she could manage, one that was bound up in a medical environment within which she was familiar and felt safe as long as she was in control. Ella was able to cry for her child, for herself and also for her mother, who she was also finally able to express her rage towards. The group held Ella while she did so.

Conclusion

The focus of this chapter is on integrating principles of intersectionality to strengthen and enhance group analytic therapy for incarcerated women with histories of serious offending and complex emotional needs. The particular value of intersectionality was identified in terms of its utility as a framework for analysing the impact of multiple marginalised identities, its origin in the lived experience of the oppressed and voiceless and in its stated robustness for holding together otherwise fragmented and dispersed aspects of a person or community.

Foulkes's group analytic construct of the matrix was considered from an inter-sectional perspective and, as such, conceptualised as an intersectional matrix. This term has been coined in an attempt to capture the impact, interplay and complex-ity involved in containing and working analytically with a considerable range and multiplicity of stigmatised and marginalised identities and the intensity of associ-ated trauma, including that which became criminogenic. The term emphasises a focus on difference and the interaction within the matrix of both complimentary and conflicting identities. It highlights the depth of thought afforded to oppression trauma and its replication within the group matrix, including as offence paralleling behaviour. The term intersectional matrix also aims to draw attention to the empiri-cal knowledge of an otherwise voiceless population and the intention of the group process to mobilise its members' agency with regard to establishing a shared narra-tive which is rooted in their lived experience and which serves to co-create a robust dynamic matrix. A representative case example has been employed to demonstrate how this approach requires considerable intersectional self-awareness and proac-tive preparation by a pair of group co-conductors.

One of the questions this paper sought to answer is whether an intersectional approach can offer an effective way to contain immense trauma, difference and complexity. The case example indicates a response to the affirmative, suffice to enable incarcerated women to find a way to be together that permits curios-ity and exploration and sufficient security to tolerate their deeper selves. Initially, this occurred through mirroring and resonance with other socially ostracised and excluded women offenders with whom, following significant intervention by co-conductors, they found the capacity to offer and receive compassion. The women used the term 'the underbelly' to essentially describe speaking openly and in their own voices about the intersection of their experiences of abuse and trauma and the abuse and trauma they themselves had perpetrated. The intersectional framework supported their narratives such that the tension between victim and perpetrator nar-ratives could be held within the group sufficiently to enable the women to find their own ways through this traumatogenic minefield, free from legal or other 'profes-sional' jargon or concepts. Importantly, doing so helped women with the process of learning about themselves in ways that shone a light on what needed to change in order for lives worth living to be salvaged from their current dire predicaments.

The role of the co-conductors is important from the perspective of Foulkes's Basic Law of Group Dynamics (Brown, 1998). Through the group, women were able to work towards processing and integrating their traumatic experiences. However, an active intervention was required by the co-conductors to prevent the women from retreating into scapegoating, perpetuating offence-paralleling phe-nomena and destructive collusion. They were required to modify the principles of monitoring of justice as described by Brown (1998). While all members were considered *equal* in terms of their humanity, members were actively encouraged to deconstruct discriminating and unjust positions taken, and as such, the principle of *impartiality* was also modified. This underlines the opinions of other authors, such as Kent (2021), Nayak (2021) and Stevenson (2020), who question Foulkes's

Basic Law of Group Dynamics and conductor positionality in the context of groups whose members have suffered considerable structural oppression. This is one of the factors to consider in a movement towards an intersectional approach to group analytic therapy. Hopefully, this chapter has raised other areas of group analytic theory and practice which are helpful to the reader working with women in criminal justice and forensic settings.

References

Aiyegbusi, A. (2020) Caught in the Racist Gaze? The Vulnerability of Black Women to Forensic Mental Health and Criminal Justice Settings. In Motz, A., Dennis, E. and Aiyegbusi, A. (eds.) *Invisible Trauma: Women, Difference and the Criminal Justice System.* London: Routledge.

Aiyegbusi, A. (2021a) The White Mirror: Face to Face with Racism in Group Analysis. Part 1 – Mainly Theory. *Group Analysis*, 54(3): 402–420.

Aiyegbusi, A. (2021b) The White Mirror: Face to Face with Racism in Group Analysis. Part 2 – Mainly Practice. *Group Analysis*, 54(3): 421–436.

Bion, W. R. (1961) *Experiences in Groups.* Oxford: Routledge.

Brown, D. G. (1998) Foulkes's Basic Law of Group Dynamics – 50 Years on: Abnormality, Injustice and the Renewal of Ethics. 22nd S.H. Foulkes Annual Lecture. *Group Analysis*, 31(4): 391–419.

Corston, J. (2007) *The Corston Report.* London: HMSO.

Crenshaw, K. (1989) Demarginalizing the Intersection of Race and Sex: A Black Feminist Critique of Anti-Discrimination Doctrine, Feminist Theory and Antiracist Politics. *University of Chicago Legal Forum*: 139–167.

Dalal, F. (1998) *Taking the Group Seriously: Towards a Post – Foulkesian Group Analytic Theory.* London: Jessica Kingsley.

Foulkes, S. H. (1975) *Group-Analytic Psychotherapy: Method and Principles.* London: Gordon & Breach.

Foulkes, S. H. (1990) *Selected Papers: Psychoanalysis and Group Analysis.* London: Karnac.

Foulkes, S. H. and Anthony, J. (1957) *Group Psychotherapy: The Psychoanalytic Approach.* London: Karnac.

Friedman, M., Rice, C. and Rinaldi, J. (2020) *Thickening Fat. Fat Bodies, Intersectionality and Social Justice.* Oxford: Routledge.

Hamad, R. (2019) *White Tears Brown Scars.* Victoria: Melbourne University Press.

Hill Collins, P. and Bilge, S. (2016) *Intersectionality.* Cambridge: Polity Press.

Inquest (2017) *Still Dying on the Inside: Examining Deaths in Women's Prisons.* https://www.inquest.org.uk/Handlers/Download.ashx?IDMF=8d39dc1d-02f7-48eb-b9ac-2c063d01656a

Kent, J. (2021) Scapegoating and the 'Angry Black Woman'. *Group Analysis*, 54(3): 354–371.

Kinouani, G. (2020) Difference, Whiteness and the Group Analytic Matrix: An Integrated Formulation. *Group Analysis*, 53(1): 60–74.

Kinouani, G. (2021) *Living While Black: The Essential Guide to Overcoming Racial Trauma.* London: Ebury Press.

Motz, A., Dennis, E. and Aiyegbusi, A. (2020) Invisible Trauma: Women, Difference and the Criminal Justice System. London: Routledge.

Nayak, S. (2020) A Response to: 'Intimate Others and the Othering of Intimates: The Gendered Psycho-Politics of the Entangled Relational' by Farhad Dalal (Dalal, 2020). *Group Analysis*, 53(4): 451–462.

Nayak, S. (2021) Black Feminist Intersectionality Is Vital to Group Analysis: Can Group Analysis Allow Outsider Ideas In? *Group Analysis*, 54(3): 337–353.

Nitzgen, D. and Hopper, E. (2017) The Concepts of the Social Unconscious and of the Matrix in the Work of S. H. Foulkes. In Hopper, E. and Weinberg, H. (eds.) *The Social Unconscious in Persons, Groups, and Societies. Volume 3: The Foundation Matrix Extended and Re-configured.* London: Karnac.

Parker, M. (2007) Repeating Patterns: Sexual Abuse and Sexual Offending. In Parker, M. (ed.) *Dynamic Security: the Democratic Therapeutic Community in Prison.* London: Jessica Kingsley, pp 189–199.

Pines, M. (2000) The Group as a Whole. In Brown, D. and Zinkin, L. (eds.) *The Psyche and the Social World: Developments in Group-Analytic Theory.* London: Jessica Kingsley, ch. 4, pp. 47–69.

Potter, H. (2015) *Intersectionality and Criminology. Disrupting and Revolutionizing Studies of Crime.* Oxford: Routledge.

Prison Reform Trust and Hibiscus Initiatives (2017) *Counted Out: Black, Asian and Minority Ethnic Women in the Criminal Justice System.* www.prisonreformtrust.org.uk/

Roberts, J. P. (1982) Foulkes' Concept of the Matrix. *Group Analysis*, 15(2): 111–126.

Scanlon, C. and Adlam, J. (2022) *Psycho-social Explorations of Trauma, Exclusion and Violence: Un-housed Minds and Inhospitable Environments.* Oxford: Routledge.

Stein, M. V. (2022) Vulnerability and Violence: Female Group Leadership, The #MeToo Movement. In Kane, Y. I., Masselink, S. M. and Weiss, A. C. (eds.) *Women, Intersectionality, and Power in Group Psychotherapy Leadership.* New York: Routledge, ch. 12, pp. 170–185.

Stevenson, S. (2020) Psychodynamic Intersectionality and the Positionality of the Group Analyst: The Tension Between Analytic Neutrality and Inter-Subjectivity. *Group Analysis*, 53(4): 498–514.

Truth, S. (1851) *Ain't I a Woman?* https://thehermitage.com/wp-content/uploads/2016/02/Sojourner-Truth_Aint-I-a-Woman_1851.pdf

Turner, D. (2021) *Intersections of Privilege and Otherness in Counselling and Psychotherapy.* Oxford: Routledge.

Chapter 2

Do Black Women's Bodies Matter in Group Analysis? Moving From Double to Intersectional Consciousness

Anthea Benjamin

I have been thinking a lot about Audre Lorde's seminal paper (2018 [1979]) 'The master's tools will never dismantle the master's house' and the work of addressing racial trauma in groups. Morgan (2021) has written about the paradox and dilemmas of whiteness within Western culture and the need to address this. We are starting to grapple with the importance of addressing whiteness, as Black people and people of coloured bodies often react to being with white bodies due to the intergenerational trauma carried in their bodies (Menakem, 2017:15). I am a believer in the importance of groups and spaces to heal and addressing the deep wounds of racism. This chapter asserts the imperative of critical intersectional conciseness and the development of a double consciousness to fully address the needs of Black and people of colour, particularly Black women. The work of groups is in crossing boundaries into the unknown, especially in light of what Menakem (2017) comments, 'when two or more unfamiliar bodies first encounter one another, each body tends to either relax in recognition or constrict in self-protection'. This struggle is more pronounced for racially minoritised members to find a home in groups, especially in holding their otherness in their skin.

Intersectionality in Groups

Foulkes and Anthony (1957:27) state, 'The first and foremost aspect with which group psychotherapists are usually concerned, and according to which they form their concepts, is that of belonging, or participation'. Group psychotherapy theory, literature and practice have mostly been developed by white men with a lack of attention to issues related to race and gender, and how this relates to emerging power dynamics in group therapy. This reinforces the idea that white people set standards of humanity by which they are bound to succeed (Dyer, 2005:12). Herein lies the precise problem that Audre Lorde makes reference to in her question, 'What does it mean when the tools of a racist patriarchy are used to examine the fruits of that same patriarchy?' Lorde's answer is, 'It means that only the most narrow perimeters of change are possible and allowable' which points to the process of (re)enactment. This is an issue when the key element of therapeutic groups is about mirroring; when this doesn't take place, it is very much like the 'still face'

DOI: 10.4324/9781003232216-3

experiment failure (Tronick et al., 1978). This 'still face' effect is often the experience of Black people and people of colour in groups where racial trauma enactments are often overlooked. Leighton (2018:21) states that understanding oppression, like symptoms of trauma, are metabolised and stored in the body, necessitates addressing oppression through the body. Therefore, group analysis needs to tend to bodies in the group setting.

Groups are about how we find our sense of self and belonging, but it is often an arduous process. These processes land on bodies both as social and interpersonal stories. The work of groups is to understand both the intra-psychic and the social as inextricably linked, without having to choose one over the other; this includes the body. Intersectionality is a helpful lens to make sense of this. Cho et al. (2013) consider intersectionality as:

An intersectional way of thinking about the problem of sameness and difference and its relation to power. This framing – conceiving of categories not as distinct but always permeated by other categories, fluid and changing, always in the process of creating and being created by dynamics of power – emphasising what intersectionality does rather than what intersectionality is.

(p. 795)

Therefore, the need to address and interrogate intersectional identities related to race and gender in therapy, particularly in groups, becomes a vital part of facilitating groups thinking about how black and brown bodies are held in these spaces. Intersectionality has its roots in Black feminist thinking in critiquing systemic power, particularly how Black women experience multiple levels of discrimination throughout society. Intersectionality has fast become a coveted framework, which is becoming a universal tool in thinking about power relations. The danger of this flatlining of power is that Black women's on-going marginalisation and oppression become obscured, as intersectionality is parachuted from its roots and becomes a tool for all. My critique is not to say intersectionality does not have something useful to offer in looking at a range of identities. But 'the shadow obscuring this black women intellectual tradition is neither accidental nor benign' (Hill Collins, 2000:3).

I have been curious about the position of Black women's bodies in group analysis. I am a Black, female, cisgender, abled-bodied psychotherapist who lives and works in London, UK. As a practitioner who was trained originally as an integrative practitioner, the emphasis was on intersubjectivity. The body, therefore, has been a clear focus for me in the attachment dance, i.e., the relational and embodied dynamic between people and conscious and unconscious communication that leads to attachments. This attachment dance, particularly for newborns and infants, is where we start to build the important building blocks of becoming a coherent self, often through mirroring processes. In group analysis, usually, we have five or more bodies together to reflect together and heal from the introjects they have consciously and unconsciously carried. This intersubjective field of experience within groups is of seeing yourself as others see you while at the same time not dissociating from the experience of how you see yourself (Bromberg, 2008:331). The problem comes when people cannot see you for yourselves but through the lens of societal and intergenerational narratives. This is a core issue for black/brown bodies and white bodies engaging in dialogue about race as they need to address their embodied privilege. For white members, this often leads to enactments of 'not knowing' or 'dissociation' in a bid to avoid the discomfort of race and racism. This painful reflection leads to a threat to self for white members, as they have not developed a double consciousness that would enable white members to hold onto a known self-image whilst opening to understanding a racialised self. These experiences come through sensory communications, permeating our skin, flesh and being.

Contextual intersectionality (Anthias, 2011) considers how I/we are socialised and positioned, and the context will constitute the figuration and how they overlap. When these intergenerational and ongoing racialised experiences are habitually not held in mind in the group, these formative and current experiences can regularly become erased by the group conductor. Our positionality determines how we experience the world and how we interpret group dynamics. One of the failures in most therapeutic modalities is the inability to consider context, the difference of being housed in an 'othered' body through a range of intersectional identities. For example, being a female, disabled and queer holds a particular embodied experience of being in the world. These identities intersect and shape a person's physical movement in the world, not often held together in group therapy in a meaningful way. Christine Sharpe (2016:15–14) talks about an aspect of Black beingness as being 'in the wake'; by this, she means 'to be occupied by the continuous and changing presence of slavery'. This intergenerational trauma is always very close to the surface in therapy groups, particularly for Black women. The messages of being inferior and caretakers for the world are important social dynamics to hold in mind for Black women to be held safely in the group setting.

Racial Trauma

Personal and societal messages that cause harm get stuck in the body and can be what brings people to group therapy to experience themselves in relationships. Foulkes comments that *projection, introjection* and *identification* are three intimately interwoven mechanisms (1990:58) that move around in group processes. I am interested in Hill Collins' (2000) ideas about how intersectionality carries an important indicator for our abilities to empathise with one another's experience of oppression or marginalisation, which enables reparative experiences. By this, Hill Collins means these othered experiences are often not understood or talked about in-depth, which can lead to a lack of attunement to members' intersectional experiences. Group members who are able to hold the interchangeable roles of perpetrator and victim become significant in this process to enable healing. These processes of victim and perpetrator move into and between bodies and are important containers of the disturbance produced from these experiences and important communications within the group. Given that groups replay experiences of privilege or marginalisation as they replicate social-historical contexts, it becomes important for us as group analysts to actively engage with these intersecting processes as they land on bodies, particularly bodies more susceptible to these projective processes. In (1994 [1903]), Du Bois described 'double consciousness' as a sense of 'always looking at oneself through the eyes of a white other' (1903:2). Therefore, group analysts need to develop more of a 'double consciousness' to see these dynamics in action.

Hillman and Ventura (1992) state, 'We've had a hundred years of psychotherapy and the world is getting worse'. He goes on to say: 'The buildings are sick, the institutions are sick, the banking systems are sick, the schools, the street – the sickness is out there' (1992:4). Our bodies are often the containers of this sickness that gets expressed in symptoms. These symptoms, i.e., weathering effects of intersectional racism, are felt within groups and are often overlooked. The term *weathering* was coined by Dr Arline Geronimus (1992), and it is a metaphor for how stress caused by everyday racism shapes or *weathers* the body. Dr Arline Geronimus states, 'In weathered populations, people and families have multiple morbidities. They can be hypertension or diabetes, depression and anxiety, joint pains, autoimmune disorders, like lupus'. Thinking about these symptoms is important because black bodies are more likely to be holding powerful projective processes in embodied ways for the group. This silencing of black bodies in general (the silencing of othered experiences and embodied experiences) leads to the complexity of oppressive practices (Kent, 2021). This is because black bodies have been socialised and become adaptive in withstanding unseen disturbances often pushed into them. Oppression and discrimination affect how we view both ourselves and the bodies we are in; it lodges in our system, skin, flesh and bones. This becomes a form of trauma that is all too often dismissed. Bodies that are positioned as non-normative identities experience significant traumatic effects, which lead to profound experiences of projection and disembodiment, which need naming and addressing. Ta-Nehisi Coates calls this level of 'disembodiment a kind of terrorism' (2015:114), and like terrorism, we need to be proactive and alert to these enactments in groups with members within these groupings. The discourse is focused on how white people can develop 'a double consciousness' to hold the intersectional experiences related to race (Du Bois, 1903). The challenge with this level of trauma is it often 'becomes a wordless story which becomes the unconscious indicators of what's safe and what's unsafe' (Menakem, 2017:8). This wordless story often lives on in our bodies and can be retrieved through attention to the bodily narrative within groups.

Bodies in Groups

White-bodied supremacy is always functioning in relation to black and brown bodies in the group setting. This operates in our thinking, in our nervous systems and in our sense of safety everywhere. Trauma is what happens to the body, and this trauma gets stuck in the body until it's addressed. So, what happens when you have a group of bodies together, all interacting with each other in groups? How can we, as group analysts, use intersectionality to better attune to the needs of traumatised bodies?

Brown states,

The bodily level is seen to be a deep level, both for the individual functioning and the group functioning. As group therapists we need to keep all our senses alert to what is going on in the bodies of individuals, the group and of ourselves.
(2006:15).

In this sense, group analysis needs to hold an intersectional lens of the bodies in groups, holding their embodied stories interwoven within treatment. These bodies often become important communication vessels for the group, which enables the deep work in the group to take place. This will include how the cultural and inter-generational narratives will come into the group through embodied states. Body-centred approaches hold the view that sensations, breath, and movement are the body's form of speech (Caldwell, 1996:4). This communication comes from the unconscious, and in listening to this important communication, we can facilitate the release of embodied trauma.

We now know that privilege and marginalisation have a profound impact on how bodies interact with their environment. Siegel's (1999) model of the window of tolerance has been a helpful model for understanding regulation in bodies. What it does not account for is that a regulated state is a form of privilege. This is because black bodies endure violence on a daily basis in the form of micro and macro aggressions and, therefore, do not have the privilege to stay or return to rested, regulated states that bodies seen as 'normal' take for granted. This is due to the unequal distribution of racial trauma laid on black and brown bodies. Bodies that are more marginalised are more likely to be operating outside of the typical ideas of the window of tolerance as they have to face more stressful experiences, which they need to adapt to. Most trauma models think about trauma work taking place once the trauma is over; with experiences such as racism, homophobia, transphobia, etc. These projective processes are ongoing and are never over, and could be known as continuous traumas. The need to be hypervigilant on multiple levels with intersectional complicity means regulation is contextual. Therefore, our work needs to be focused on group members' contexts and how, due to intersectional positioning, not all bodies experience the same thing, even if, on a biological level, we are ultimately the same.

Language in Groups

Part of therapy is the re-humanisation process of dehumanised aspects of self often held in the stereotype. Stereotypes are held and communicated in language through verbal and non-verbal communication. This needs to apply also to bodies that have been fundamentally dehumanised for who they are and the bodies they occupy.

Many Black women in groups become labelled as *'the angry Black woman'*, *'Superwoman'* or *'the mammie'*. Black women are susceptible to the projective processes which position them and are circumscribed in society. This stereotyping gets in the way of being experienced as real and becomes a socialisation process of either being assimilated into group norms or becoming misunderstood or marginalised. This can result in silencing within the group context and becomes a tension for Black women. We live in cultures built on colonialism, patriarchy, homophobia, transphobia, etc. Layton and Leavy-Sperounis (2020:xvii) talk about fighting 'a memoryless present'. Layton goes on to say:

> *The dangerous decontextualising of human experience, shuts down a collective ability to think, and inhibit a collective capacity to mourn.*
>
> (2020:xvii)

With an intersectional lens, the work of the group would be to find the shared language to acknowledge the shared culture we inhabit, where a collective mourning can be facilitated. For many people coming to therapy, the work is to mourn what was never received or lost and to come to terms with this loss with some hope for what they can open up to in the here and now. Sharpe (2016:11) speaks to the difficulty of thinking about slavery and its afterlife, which is likely to be an important embodied experience for members of the Black community. She goes on to say:

> *Black people become the carriers of terror, terrors embodiment, and not the primary objects of terrors multiple enactments, the ground of terror's possibility globally.*
>
> (2016:15)

These phenomena exist in group work, but the difficulty is to think about the ongoing impact of intergeneration trauma, such as slavery, because of the likely intergenerational complicity in other group members, even when it enters the room. This is also due to internalised derogative messages about blackness. There is a lot to blackness, and within this, there are a range of intersectional identities.

> *Alex, 36, is a non-binary Black person. There has been an ongoing process between group members referring to Alex as 'she' rather than their real embodied identity as 'them' and 'they'. This has been taking place for months. The group is challenged to consider their own discomfort about Alex's transition to non-binary and how the struggle to refer to their gender pronouns may be a form of passive aggression about group members' difficulties with Alex's transition. When this is raised, the group falls into shame, dismissing their feelings about the difficulty with Alex transitioning. Alex raises this as not the first time they have experienced their identity dismissed as the group often overlooks their race. The group is asked to consider what gets re-enacted with Alex in the group. A member talks about how scary they experience Alex*

as being and refers to shortness of breath around them and finding it hard to talk. The group responds to this group member's struggles with Alex. Alex sits in silence as the group refers to them as a third person and finally finds their voice to express their distress in holding microaggressions from the group and becoming more silent as they are picking up the unconscious communication from the group about difficulties about their difference. Alex goes on to talk about their experiences outside the group where people often ignore their difference, or they get positioned as scary, and how painful this form of erasure is. Alex then talks about their felt sense of safety in the group being minimal and needing to protect themselves by keeping themselves separate. The group falls into a long silence. Alex goes on to say they are considering if it is best to be in a group with more diverse group members and goes silent. One member bravely names her discomfort and worries about sharing her discomfort, and is terrified of 'getting it wrong' and 'saying the wrong thing'. Slowly, the group discusses how, whether they name their prejudices or not, they have a visceral impact on bodies in the group, particularly on Alex. This brings up distress in Alex as they have had to deal with people's passive aggression about their identities most of their life. One member talks about finding it difficult to breathe in the group and links this to Alex's experience. Alex talks about the desire to be in a body and a skin that is accepted and wants to be more able to breathe authentically, but it is hard to breathe in this group and places a hand on their chest briefly. The analyst asks Alex to keep their hand on their chest and to notice what comes up. The group begins a collective holding of breath, noticing themselves. Members, in different ways, shift or move in their chairs, almost like trying to find more room for their bodies. The analyst comments on the challenge of not having their experience fully mirrored in the group and the distress and confusion this evokes. The group slowly starts to think about how they can be brave and talk about their conflicted feelings and own their biased attitudes in the group, enacting painful normative communications to each other in not being able to remember their pronouns or address race.

The work of a group is to find a shared language from which to meet, to find ways to be with what is not understood and find a way to be with each other. This language is not just the spoken word but includes sensations, impulses, images, feelings, etc. This is particularly interesting to me in terms of what the cultural norms have been about vulnerability and the historical processes of disavowal and projection placed on certain bodies. The concept of a cultural norm, having the same language and the hierarchy of power raises a number of issues. Cultural norms of how to meet others often create barriers in assumptions about which norms will be privileged and followed. This is also true in terms of how bodies are experienced and perceived, such as which bodies are considered vulnerable and need protecting, which bodies are considered dangerous and to be wary of and which are held within a cultural and contextual context.

Opening to the Process

Foulkes described the 'matrix' of the group as a 'dynamically interrelated network – the psychic fabric of the total group' (Foulkes and Anthony, 1957:255). In developing this, the group members need to open themselves to the group and allow themselves to be known. This is particularly challenging when you have learned to armour yourselves due to micro and macro aggressions, which often are unseen or dismissed. Opening up becomes a minefield and potentially something that puts black and brown group members at more risk of harm. Foulkes talks about the restoration of disturbed communication and this being the operational basis of all group therapy. The challenge is when there is no restoration, as intersectional microaggressions are not seen or heard due to people's own context and limited experience. This can leave Black women, particularly those holding multiple marginalised intersectional identities, isolated and alienated. This can, therefore, reinforce societal experiences and often lead to not opening up, silencing and or splitting off parts of self in order to belong, feel safe and survive the experience of the group setting.

Gendlin (1978) talks about 'felt sense', which is a deepening into self through an inter-and intra-psychic experience of self and other. This includes working with conflicted thoughts and feelings about self and others. Bodies unconsciously contract and relax with each other, but often, these processes are not openly named in groups. Time given to body processes would enable the group to engage with body narratives that inhabit our socialised self. This has been particularly powerful when members have talked about feelings embodied which they don't have words for in relation to other members in the group, and it has been important to make space for and to keep coming back to what Foulkes would refer to as autistic communication (1964:68) to understand the different levels of communications taking place in the group between members. George Yancy writes, there is a peculiarity in experiencing one's body as a thing *confiscated* yet without the evidence of physical chains (2008). This can often be communicated in groups through microaggressions, which are small, consistent and deliberate messages, often unconsciously communicated to marginalised bodies. The cumulative impact of these intersectional assaults is a huge cost when not picked up. Resmaa Menken talks about there being two types of pain: clean pain and dirty pain. Clean pain is the process of metabolising pain through the body by slowing things down and allowing the process to be experienced more by referencing the process within bodies (2017:19). By moving the process between thinking and processing in the body, we are staying more fully with important trauma reactions. This allows opportunities for settling within the nervous system and creates more space in the individual and collective systems to hold each other and co-regulate in more depth. Dirty pain is the avoidance, blaming processes and denial of harm caused between members. These processes become enactments of people's cultural and historical contexts, and the activation of intergenerational trauma becomes reinforced and amplified.

> *Josey is a Black woman, 41, working-class, of Caribbean descent, who has been a friendly, warm and gregarious member of a group. Since the BLM movement,*

she has become overwhelmed with traumatic memories of her experiences of racism. She starts to open up about these experiences in more depth and names her difficulty bringing these themes to a mixed group. The group members are thoughtful but can only engage with the conversation by placing all the difficulty out there in the world and cannot pick up anything about the difficulty that clearly exists within the group where she is not feeling safe enough to bring these experiences in. The group analyst wondered about the intersectional relationship between race and class and how these intersectional identities affect her both in the world and in the group. She shares her experience as a Black working-class woman of having to make herself 'safe or useful' and how she has to overcompensate to protect herself from being perceived as 'the angry Black woman'. An exploration develops about how she is often dominant in the group in helping others and how her vulnerability is often unseen. The group discusses whose vulnerability is seen and how white women's tears are privileged in the group as 'real' vulnerability. This recognition wakes Josey up, and she talks about the number of times she has been extremely vulnerable in the group and has shed a tear, but somehow, her tears are ignored. The group goes silent. The group is slowly encouraged to talk about how white women's tears have become the 'standard of humanity', *about their own projections onto Josey and to take back their intersectional biases towards her, which she has unconsciously picked up, resulting in her assuming a role of 'the mammie (caretaker)' both in the group and in her wider context. Josey silently sheds tears, and the group reflects on her silent tears as a reflection of the previous erasure of her pain and of her in the group. This leads to a cathartic process of deep breathing, which has a ripple effect on other bodies in the group alongside her.*

Resmaa Menakem talks about trauma not only occurring in the individual but as a contagious disease that moves between bodies (2017:37). The collective group need to be open to this, bear witness and hold the depth and breadth of historical trauma when shared, which is likely to arouse each member's own intergenerational resonance in relation to their own trauma. In this way, it can be like a domino effect that can be a delicate yet powerful group experience. Part of this ripple effect is the movement between victim and perpetrator states depending on a member's 'position' and historical context. The temporal and spatial dimensions of intersectionality need to be linked both to the outside, historical context and to the here and now, how these roles and positions are mirrored in the group. In these moments, reparative opportunities appear. The group then comes into its own as mother in birthing new experiences, which can feel like new skin and new bodied experiences where members can be seen in their fullness.

Conclusion

Addressing the traumatising cultural messages which lay on, and in, the bodies of Black women, in particular, with much weight, requires us to centralise the body-mind connection. This requires us to develop a critical intersectional consciousness, which would mean acknowledging the intersectional links between trauma, oppression, power, privilege and the range of historical inequalities operating in all social relationships. Foulkes (1990:152–156) talks about isolation and alienation being the problem of our time and how groups are supportive of reducing this sense of alienation. Foulkes felt groups bring the problems back to where they belong, in the community, so the task in groups is to support Black women to bring the problems projected onto them back to the group where they belong . . . in the community. In engaging with intersectionality in group analysis, we can address normative assumptions in working with Black women in groups in using additional tools to the existing 'master tools' Lorde referred to, to enable more inclusive practice. Intersectionality enables us to challenge the pattern of embodied projective processes into black bodies, and the group analyst's vital role is to support the group in developing a double consciousness. This is not a constant state but a reiterative circular experience of coming more into wholeness and integrating intersectional identities. The group conductor needs to have done and continue to do their own work on their own intersectional identities, as the group as a whole will be reflecting the conductor's own fragmentation. This is because groups reflect the conductor's own unprocessed and processed parts of their psyche. It is here where we can expand the frame beyond the master's tools so that we can better address the historical and ongoing harm being done to the marginalised bodies of Black women. This is fundamental and necessary for group work that is genuinely inclusive and reparative for all members of a group and for society as a whole.

References

Anthias, F. (2011) Intersections and Translocations: New Paradigms for Thinking About Cultural Diversity and Social Identities. *European Educational Research Journal*, 10(2): 204–217.

Bromberg, P. (2008) Shrinking the Tsunami: Affect Regulation, Dissociation, and the Shadow of the Flood. *Contemporary Psychoanalysis*, 44(3): 329–350.

Caldwell, C. (1996) *Getting Our Bodies Back: Recovery, Healing and Transformation Through Body-Centred Psychotherapy*. Colorado: Shambhala Publications.

Cho, S., Crenshaw, K. W. and McCall, L. (2013) Toward a Field of Intersectionality Studies: Theory, Applications, and Praxis. *Signs*, 38(4): 785–810.

Coates, T-N. (2015) Between the World and Me. New York: Random House.

Du Bois, W. E. B. (1994 [1903]) *The Souls of Black Folk*. New York: Dover Publications, Inc.

Dyer, R. (2005) The Matter of Whiteness. In Rothenberg, P. S. (ed.) *White Privilege: Essential Readings on the Other Side of Racism*. New York: Worth Publishers, pp. 9–17.

Foulkes, S. H. (1964) *Therapeutic Group Analysis*. London: Karnac Books.

Foulkes, S. H. (1990) *Selected Papers: Psychoanalysis and Group Analysis*. London: Karnac.

Foulkes, S. H. and Anthony, E. J. (1957) *Group Psychotherapy: The Psychoanalytic Approach*. London: Karnac.

Gendlin, E. (1978) *Focusing*. New York, NY: Bantam Dell.

Geronimus, A. T. (1992) The Weathering Hypothesis and the Health of African-American Women and Infants: Evidence and Speculations. *Ethnicity & Disease*, 2(3): 207–221.

Hill Collins, P. (2000) *Black Feminist Thought: Knowledge, Consciousness, and the Politics of Empowerment*, 2nd ed. London: Routledge.

Hillman, J. and Ventura, M. (1992) We've Had a Hundred Years of Psychotherapy – And the World's Getting Worse. New York: HarperCollins.

Kent, J. (2021) Scapegoating and the 'angry black woman'. *Group Analysis*, 54(3), 354–371.

Layton, L. and Leavy-Sperounis, M. (2020) *Towards a Social Psychoanalysis: Culture, Character and Normative Unconscious Processes*. London: Routledge.

Leighton, L. B. (2018) The Trauma of Oppression: A Somatic Perspective. In Caldwell, C. and Leighton, L. B. (ed.) Oppression and the Body: Roots, Resistance and Resolution. Berkeley, CA: North Atlantic Books, pp. 17–30.

Lorde, A. (2018 [1979]) The Master's Tools Will Never Dismantle the Master's House. London: Penguin Classics.

Martinez, J. (2020) The major health ramifications of racial "weathering" on Black people. Well + Good. Available at: https://www.wellandgood.com/what-is-weathering/ (Accessed 2024 Jan 10)

Menakem, R. (2017) *My Grandmother's Hands: Racialised Trauma and the Pathways to Mending Our Hearts and Bodies*. Las Vegas, NV: Central Recovery Press.

Morgan, H. (2021) Whiteness: A Problem for Our Times. *British Journal of Psychotherapy*, 37: 469–483.

Sharpe, C. (2016) *In the Wake: On Blackness and Being*. Durham, NC: Duke University Press.

Siegel, D. J. (1999) *The Developing Mind*. New York: Guilford.

Tronick, E., Als, H., Adamson, L., Wise, S. and Brazelton, T. B. (1978) The Infant's Response to Entrapment between Contradictory Messages in Face-to-Face Interaction. *Journal of American Academy of Child Psychiatry*, 17: 1–13.

Yancy, G. (2008) Elevators, Social Spaces and Racism: A Philosophical Analysis. Philosophy and Social Criticism, 34(8): 843–876.

Chapter 3

The Body of the Group

Sexuality, Transgender, and Group Polyphony[1]

Daniel Anderson

Sexuality and gender are arguably invisible (or at least less visible) products of identity. The body, generally hidden under clothing, reveals itself through contour, behaviour, and imagination. Gendered clothing offers little evidence of the body underneath. Sexuality and gender require an extra effort within language to state a position or 'come out' to use a colloquialism. For the sake of clarity, I shall briefly state mine as an author working alongside a group of authors in this book on intersectionality: I am a gay, white, and cis-gendered man. Even this revelation is a curious act when considered alongside race where the tendency is (or has been) less inclined to state race so definitively. Skin colour provides its own bodily statement but also its own projective screen onto which the minds of others distort themselves and the recipient. I am also mindful that once typed and published, it is a statement by me that is not easily reversed. Perhaps here, there is some solidarity for me with race, where skin colour, in general, is equally difficult to hide.

This chapter will specifically address sexuality and (trans)gender in relation to group analysis and their relationship to other aspects of social difference, such as the body, race, class, and religion. I would like to introduce two terms to help me formulate my response to intersectionality, and that also enables a dialogue between group analysis and queer theory: the 'field imaginary' and figuration. But first, a polemic statement: group analysis has failed to fully articulate the sexual and gender minorities beyond heteronormativity and psychopathology. However, as I shall argue, this will probably be helpful to its development in that it has adroitly (and accidentally) situated itself as a field domain within lack and failure that is crucial for fully appreciating any political project. The analytic group is a means to contain and mobilise the failure of language and ideas that are integral to understanding the analytic group. By lack, I am referring to an absence of discourse such that there is a gap in understanding and speech. Similarly, by failure, I am referring to how knowledge changes and alters within the iterative experience of being in an analytic group such that the meaning of the original word or term fails to represent what it used to represent. Failure can also mean a lack, however, in that it implies a conscious or unconscious neglect. Either way, the group can function as a space and time to contain the dynamics of absence and failure that otherwise can become destructive.

DOI: 10.4324/9781003232216-4

Group analysis and group analysts are, however, not beyond politics and history and the subjective experience of those attending analytic groups, whatever their sexual, gender, and other such intersectional identifications. They are as prone to prejudices such as racism, homophobia, and transphobia, consciously and unconsciously, as anyone else. The problem is that the field domain of group analysis is bound to historical accounts of the relationship between homosexuality and psychoanalysis, resulting in group analysis historically referring to non-normative sexualities and genders as being reduced to perversion and developmental arrest or grossly reduced to a singular category of identity.

However, this statement of mine should not ignore work that has occurred recently within group analysis. For example, Watson (2005) suggests that being queer is akin to being like someone in therapy who is in a state of flux and is challenging boundaries and definitions. Likewise, Bacha (2005) proposes that sexuality can be broken down into identity, desire, and gender. By doing so, Bacha argues that we see the inherent instability of identity based around sexuality. Bacha further proposes that being in an analytic group could be seen as a queer experience in itself in that it is an attempt to deconstruct identity through dialogue. What exactly is meant by the term queer in this regard is unclear and may be taken for granted.

Notwithstanding this statement of mine, it is the embodiment of group analytic theory within a contained gendered and sexualised analytic group that has profound implications for sexuality and gender as enabled by the analytic group's potential to simultaneously contain multiple and often contradictory thoughts and feelings. I have deliberately bracketed the notions of asexuality and agender alongside sexuality and gender. It is a partial refrain by me that I hope holds a tension between the political task of addressing such identities and maintaining a de-politicised position that I argue is at the core of the group analytic task. By doing so, I shall demonstrate the capacity of group analysis to potentially finely balance and contain political and apolitical tasks when considering sexuality and gender and their interactions with other identifications. The two previously mentioned terms will aid me: the 'field imaginary' and figuration. Before I explicate these processes using film and clinical vignette material, I would like to set the scene a little by briefly reviewing the political field that group analysis has come from.

Where Have We Come From?

I am not going to attempt a history of sexuality and gender in group analysis or, indeed, in psychoanalysis. Space here is an issue, but I am also mindful that I am interested in decentring the power of the author. Who am I to consider myself as a narrator of that history, and what are the consequences to the reader and to the narrative if I were to do so? Instead, I shall highlight what I consider to be the lowest point of that history where classical psychoanalysis forgot that it was meant to be a subject that aided its patients rather than traumatised them. I use the term 'trauma' deliberately here. Much has been written about the apparently pathological nature of the 'homosexual'. Very little has turned this around to consider the pathology-inducing nature of the discourse within certain schools of psychoanalysis surrounding the 'homosexual' and the 'pervert' that subsequently results in traumatising the subject. The prolific nature of such writings and their pervasive existence within Western society at least has become akin to a 'death by a thousand cuts'. Fear of violence and the dread of the unexpected and often covert nature of discrimination mean that many of those who identify as a sexual or gender minority have had their developmental years tainted by avoidance, vigilance, and runaway fantasies of being victimised for being 'other'. In this context, it is no wonder that the 'closet' appeared. I am also mindful that the literature had historically made little if no reference to any notion of sexuality and colour. It has remained a white literature dominated by middle-class men.

I also use the term 'death by a thousand cuts' deliberately. Seldom is the trauma a singular 'gay-bashing' event that we might hear about in the news. Often, it is also the insidious and cumulative effects of multiple insults. A flick through some of the core writings of group analysis by its originator, Siegmund Foulkes, will quickly reveal such 'cuts', and it is imperative that the authors or trainers of group analysis root out such insults to prevent these 'cuts' becoming a 'death'. I do not write this statement as being akin to 'throwing the baby out with the bath water'. A historical perspective is important to note movement and change, but it must be given a perspective in time and space for criticism and response.

As an example, here is a period of psychoanalytic time: the "Conservative Developments". This period between 1948 and 1963 saw a proliferation of psychoanalytic writing on homosexuality that "was characterized by an increasingly moralistic tone and a growing emphasis on conventional social values" (Lewes, 1995:128). One of the most prolific writers was Edmond Bergler (1947, 1948, 1951, 1956), whose blatant attack on homosexuality was nothing short of abusive: "Homosexuality is not the 'way of life' these sick people gratuitously assume it to be, but a neurotic distortion of the total personality" (Bergler, 1956:9). Bergler (1956) termed homosexuality a 'disease' and concluded that:

> *there are no healthy homosexuals*. The entire personality structure of the homosexual is pervaded by the *unconscious* wish to suffer; this wish is gratified by self-created *trouble-making*. This "injustice-collecting" (technically called psychic masochism) is conveniently deposited in the external difficulties confronting the homosexual. If they were to be removed – and in some circles in large cities they have been virtually removed – the homosexual would still be an emotionally sick person.
>
> (Bergler, 1956:9, original italics)

I recognise that by writing in this way as a gay, white, cis-gender man, I may be fulfilling exactly what Bergler was describing here. As Bergler stated, "The homosexual of either sex believes that his (sic) trouble stems from the 'unreasonable attitude' of the environment" (Bergler, 1956:9). There is an irony to this statement by Bergler that misgenders all 'homosexuals' as men, despite the reference to "either sex", and yet he advocates the alternative position that their "troubles" do not stem from the "'unreasonable attitude' of the environment". Bergler goes further to propose that homosexuality can be 'cured' and that the failure to 'cure' homosexuality is, of course, the fault of the 'homosexual': "All this [homosexuality] can be remedied by information combined with treatment, *provided the prospective patient really wants to change*" (Bergler, 1956:10, original italics).

Perhaps I am 'trouble-making' by challenging the hegemony through my 'injustice-collecting'. I do accept some of these terms (because there are injustices that need naming, and it takes a certain degree of narcissism to publish), but I also would like to turn it around; the terms create themselves. My response to the quote indirectly affirms the content of the quotes and their apparent truth – not because they are true but because they are offensive. Irrespective of what is apparently being 'acted out', as some might argue, I stand by my statements because I feel I must; otherwise, I become a victim of their shaming. Most people who identify as a sexual or gender minority, in my experience, have been told enough times they are not wanted, or they are sick, and I have a hope in group analysis that it has the will and ability to move past such oppression and is honest enough to recognise its past complicity and harm.

Field Imaginary

Moving back to failure, the failure of ideas is necessary and useful because it allows the space and time for new ideas to grow and for discourse to move beyond. Stacey (2015) mobilises the term field imaginary to discuss subjects who are motivated by the political desire for social justice in relation to gender and sexuality by tracking the affective investment and subsequent attachment into discursive formations by those subjects in such an intense and overinvested manner that "their disappointments and failures are almost built into their gestures" (p. 47). Furthermore, Stacey argues that such disappointments and failures are built into the founding gestures of the desire for social justice in the field imaginaries such that the identity knowledge produced will necessarily fail to deliver what may be promised by such endeavours. The crucial aspect to consider is that we cannot extricate ourselves, in terms of our own desires, from identity knowledge production and the eventual failure of identity knowledge within these political projects. Our own personal disappointments and failures, as fantasies, become projected and enacted through the project of the field imaginary directly because they were present, consciously or not, at the foundation of such epistemology such that they operate to structure such knowledge (Stacey, 2015).

Likewise, Freudian and Kleinian psychoanalysis has failed to articulate a non-pathologising and non-identity-based view of non-normative sexualities and genders. For group analysis, which thankfully has never had its own theory of psycho-sexuality, this failure permits a potentiality to dislocate the body from gender, desire, sex, and sexuality by virtue of the fact that the politics of such terms were (arguably, at least directly) never part of its inception. The converse is true for psychoanalysis, which arguably had sexuality at the forefront of its first patient, Anna O (Breuer and Freud, 1955 [1895]). I caution against idealising group analysis, however, in that it does fail with sexuality by its reification of sexuality and gender as identities through which the self can be organised. Nonetheless, the potential emphasis on the body within group analysis enables a view of sexuality that cannot be localised within one body but can also be within the collective body of the group. This moves sexuality from an intrapsychic event to an interpersonal process, with a subsequent expansion of language that emphasises the symbolic nature of sexuality rather than solely a biological expression of a drive. Meaning is generated through this verbalised form of desire, and, as such, sexuality becomes a social phenomenon. The next section on figuration will help to explicate this idea.

Figurations

As a cautionary note regarding failure, the lack can also be just as discriminatory as presence. Both involve potential prejudice through the respective passive or active positions. I shall shift the focus now towards the idea of active presence. To further introduce the intersectionality of some aspects of queer theory with group analytic theory, I also offer the term figuration as a means to start this dialogue. Figuration is also a term that features in both feminism and group analysis (and specifically in relation to Norbert Elias, as an original founder of group analysis). Haraway's (1991) feminist account of figuration relies on the construction of an imagined consciousness and an apprehended oppression. Haraway's presentation of the figuration of the cyborg brought about a dialogue between technoscience and feminism as a means to understand a political coalition that ordinarily had not existed before. It challenged the typical presentation of the self-other, and so enabled considerations of social networks (or kinship-network to use Haraway's term) that highlighted connections that otherwise do not fit typical Western dichotomies. In this manner, the subject is not self-creating but emerges through relating in such a way that neither subject existed before the relating act and that the relating is never complete (Bastian, 2006). The point to emphasise here is that intersectional figurations are always becoming and are never complete, an important point given the critiques of intersectionality as a reductive and limited framework (Nayak, 2014).

The figures of the figuration become a point of reference whereby meanings of relating coalesce in new, atypical, and contradictory ways. The figuration is, therefore, not static but dynamic as it emerges through shifting meanings that do not try to resolve themselves and, indeed, often remain conflicting. By doing so, figurations display gaps in knowledge and permit an alternative way of perceiving and orienting oneself that ordinarily is not possible. An important aspect of this technique is that of enjoyment such that serious play "guards against the possibility of becoming too attached to one's ideas, too arrogant, or of taking oneself too seriously" (Bastian, 2006:4). In this sense, figurations are creative experiences that disrupt the idea that language and social practices are static phenomena.

In a similar vein to Haraway, Norbert Elias tried to consider a new language that went beyond the individual-society dichotomy, arguing that this polarisation is contingent on this moment of history. It is the outcome of this 'civilising process', as Elias termed it, which has transformed not only the structure of society but the personality itself (Elias, 1994). Elias suggested that people make up webs of inter-dependence of figurations of many kinds, characterised by power balances of many sorts, such as family, school, state, and so forth. There are two points to emphasise in these discussions of figuration; first, Haraway's use of gaps in knowledge, and second, Elias's notion of figuration permitting a move beyond existing language. The subsequent film and clinical vignette examples will help to articulate these two positions regarding figurations by bringing group analysis and feminist queer theory into the conversation. Group analytic theory enables gaps and failures in language and the creation of new language, which has important implications for sexuality and gender as well as other categories of difference.

An Example: *The Boys in the Band*

Before using some fabricated clinical examples, I would like to exemplify these notions using an example from theatre and film. *The Boys in the Band* is a 1970 American drama film directed by William Friedkin, having been adapted from the original screenplay written by Mart Crowley. It is probably one of the first-ever films from America to depict the contemporary lives of a group of Western gay men. The film offers the opportunity to explore what potentially happens when a group of men identifying as gay but of different races, expressions of gender, and religions is interrupted by the arrival of someone different, in this case, an apparently straight white man. The film offers a trope of what happens when heteronormative society is interrupted by the arrival of queerness. The difference from the norm, of course, does not have to be around sexuality but could be about gender, race, or class, to name a few. It may not be a perfect example, given its male and Western dominance, but it nonetheless appropriately sets the scene.

Sedgwick (1990) likens queer to concepts such as possibilities, gaps, disso-nances, lapses in meaning, and excesses of meaning when sexuality and gender are not considered monolithically. However, Sedgwick also notes that queer could also refer to same-sex sexual object choice, whether organised around an intersectional crisscrossing of definitions or not. In this sense, queer is historical and political seeking to subvert and take a stance against heteronormativity. Finally, Sedgwick proposes a third use of the term queer along an axis that is separate from sexuality and gender and which situates queer alongside race, ethnicity, and postcolonialism as a form of discourse that is identity fracturing. The implications of Sedgwick's definitions of 'queer' as subversive and identity fracturing are significant within a group analytic process that can contain disruptive notions of lack, gaps, and failure.

Set in an Upper East Side apartment in New York in the late 1960s, it depicts Michael as the main protagonist, preparing to host a birthday party for his Jewish friend Harold. His friend Donald, who has recently moved from the city and is undergoing psychoanalysis, aids Michael, a Catholic and a writer recovering from alcoholism, in the preparation for the party. Michael receives an unexpected call from an old college friend called Alan with a request to see Michael urgently. The guests gradually arrive for the party. Emory is caricatured as a white, effeminate, flamboyant interior decorator. Bernard is a quiet and reserved black sales assistant in a bookshop. Hank and Larry are a white couple. Hank is going through a divorce from his wife, and Larry likes to sleep with other guys. After informing his guests that Alan, a straight white man, will be calling round, he asks his guests to appear less obviously 'gay'. Later, Alan calls again to say he no longer needs to come round, but then unexpectedly appears and interrupts the party.

Before Alan arrives, a young male hustler known by the name 'Cowboy' appears at the door, having been rented for the night by Michael as a 'gift' to Harold. Tensions mount as the gay men become increasingly curious about Alan and his reasons for being there. This culminates in Alan assaulting Emory after receiving a number of taunts from Emory. Harold finally makes his appearance in the middle of the brawl. As the guests become increasingly drunk, including Michael, who has now broken his previous sobriety, tensions and desires continue to escalate. The party shifts from the relative open-air and light feeling of the large balcony of the apartment to a much more sultry and dystopian experience in the lounge after a thunderstorm and heavy downpour force them inside.

Michael instigates a telephone game whereby each guest must call the one true person they believe they have loved and tell them so. As each guest makes the call, old heart-breaks, lovers, and their feelings re-surface. Bernard and Emory both immediately regret making their calls. Hank and Larry call each other through two separate lines in the apartment. Michael's plan to 'out' Alan, however, whom he presumes is at the party to reveal his 'closeted' self, does not go well. Alan calls his wife instead of his presumed ex-male lover from college, whom Michael believed he would call. As the party comes to an end, Michael consequently collapses into a fit of self-loathing and guilt about his sexuality and decides to attend midnight mass at his local Catholic church.

The film is a complex intersectional trope of how a group of an apparently singular identity is perforated by the unexpected addition of a different identity. It results in either the incorporation or rejection of the 'other' and also the projection of various hurts and their associated feelings of revenge onto the 'other'. It also represents various intersections between race, gender, and religion, to name a few, that become greater than the sum of its parts in the mix. There is an undercurrent of mental illness as seen through mental anguish, alcoholism, drug use, and psychoanalysis. There are also moralistic undertones, as seen through Hank divorcing his wife, Larry sleeping with other guys despite being with Hank, and Harold going off with a rent boy.

The party scene, however, is punctured by the unexpected telephone call from Alan, who telephones in distress and asks to come round. It is uncertain why he is in distress, but he desires contact and solace with his friend Michael. A subsequent telephone call to cancel this request and then his unexpected appearance at the door anyway, adds to the tension as seen through the visible relief from the guests of not having to pretend to be straight, especially as he walks in on the men flamboyantly dancing. Speaking group analytically, Alan becomes the location of difference for the group and, later, the location of its disturbance. The function of this location of disturbance might be named as a group defence against the intersectional weight of difference.

There is a subversion of identity whereby the group of gay men perverts their sexual identities into trying to 'act' straight but also attacks that perversion by deliberately 'slipping up' and acting queer. Michael, the main protagonist, is, of course, naturally curious about why he is at his apartment. Alan, however, refuses to put this desire into language, and in that sense, he remains unknown throughout the film in that his desire refuses symbolisation into language; his nameless desire remains devoid of meaning.

Michael seems convinced that he has come round to 'come out' and have sex. He instigates a game as a way, perhaps, of putting into language his assumed desire. The game involves telephoning the one person each man has loved and telling that person, 'I love you'. One by one, each man does this to devastating effect, whereby each man succumbs to the tragedy of his loveless state of being. When it comes to Alan, however, Michael assumes he will phone an ex-college friend with whom Michael is convinced Alan had a sexual affair. However, Alan unexpectedly telephones his wife and tells her he loves her.

In this moment, all the assumed desire and attempts to put that desire into language by the protagonist abruptly ends. He realises that his attempt to translate his desire into love (or at least the erotic by projecting it onto Alan) has been perverted into translating his desire into hate and introjected. By doing so, he realises his own self-loathing, loneliness, and destructiveness. Alan leaves having affirmed his 'heterosexuality' through the others witnessing him confirming his love for his wife, although it remains within the realm of the unknown why it was he phoned Michael in distress and came to the apartment at all. In this sense, the figurations in the film represent a triumph for heteronormativity in that the straight man can affirm his heterosexuality within the territory of the group of gay men, but it also remains mysterious as to what it is he wishes by his refusal to engage into their projected wishes. In the end, none of the attendees seem satisfied by their strict adherence to their personal individual tropes of identity.

The nameless desire comes to represent a lack-in-being, and that contact is needed to fill that lack. The telephone game was perhaps an attempt to translate unconscious desire into the language of the matrix of this group of men. For the other men who engaged in this game, including the protagonist, this did allow the bringing into language many unconscious aspects of shame, guilt, and hate. Many of the men bring such feelings into a dialogue of difference, such as their experiences of growing up feeling sexually different, or into differences around religion, class, morality, and race, for example.

Before this game was instigated, however, there was also a moment where this 'straight' man was essentially forced into a position of naming his desire to the others, which fails dramatically. This occurs around the charade of pretending they were straight and this charade failing. Emory, as a particularly effeminate gay man who was defiantly exaggerating this disruption of gender normativities, tries to assert his sexual desire onto Alan, which is consequently refused by Alan. This is an important scene of fantasy; the gay men imagine that their desire was indeed his desire that was projected onto him. However, Alan refuses it; their desire becomes thwarted and disavowed. An attempt to love instantly flips into hate, and subsequent violence ensues. Their attempt at putting into language their desire for him and his refusal to engage in that language results in the telephone game being constructed as an attempt to bring the naming of that desire into the group matrix. The others, however, could not accept Alan's refusal of this, which changes the matrix from an exclusive and apparently singular identity (homosexuality) into one of multifarious and intersectional sexualities and other such categories.

The subsequent violence is a reminder that relinquishing such positions is a two-way process that requires accommodation and engagement by all. It comes with potential risk as the power of the group moves from the dominant sexuality to include minority sexuality with the subsequent and historical hurts and traumas directed towards Alan as the handsome, healthy, white, masculine-looking man who apparently has no need to question his sexuality. The first attempt to relinquish a position (but without verbalising desire in language) fails. However, the second attempt does seem more successful – just not the way the group had hoped or expected. It results in an exposure of their own desires, longings, and histories, including their heterophobia and homophobia.

The Analytic Group

Moving past a film as a trope for the intersectional dynamics of groups, I will now consider some of these ideas in the clinical analytic group as an intersectional figuration for considering and containing the crisscrossing of language related to sexuality and gender. Attendees of analytic groups can become able to learn new, multiple, and sometimes contradictory versions of themselves and each other, and crucially, can learn to live with all of them simultaneously. Such a process does not abandon identity but celebrates the potential multiplicity of identities. However, this is not a simple process and involves disparities, memories, transferences, and memories, to name a few. For example, the following fictional vignette explores the language of sexuality and the response to words being forced upon others:

Joanne talks about her neighbours, a lesbian couple next door, one of whom she described as being "the butch one", and the other "the femme one". She also spoke about a man whom she described as being "really gay". The group challenges her use of language to understand what these terms mean. In response, Alan becomes angry at Joanne, saying it was not for her to decide what sort of gay man he is. Later in the session, he comments on his anger – it was like being at home with his mum, who would say being gay is unnatural.

I also offer this second vignette as a further example, but this time related more to transgender than sexuality:

> *Sarah, a trans-woman, revealed she had had an argument with a friend and called her a "cunt". I found this to be a curious pejorative term for a trans-woman to use, and I asked why she had angrily mocked the vagina when she so desperately craved one. Sarah found that hard to answer but knew she just felt blind rage, and it had frightened her. The group took up this fear of rage into the group space itself and used it to wonder what aggression they feared by saying the wrong thing to each other.*

In the analytic group, there are questions about what is being witnessed by the others and its role. The analytic group can seem like it wants to have the capacity to consider all identities, but often, it can openly struggle with knowing how to contain the subsequent feelings for fear of getting it wrong and making it worse. Crucially, this is not about doubting the feelings of sexuality and gender identities as if they were some types of psychopathology in need of correction. It is more about trying to make some meaning out of such categories and the shame that may accompany them, and it can also come to represent the pain of change for the whole group. Group analysis uses the terms 'scapegoating' and 'location of disturbance' to consider the group-as-a-whole process to prevent one member from doing the work for them all. These terms also apply to the other group members who equally experience various painful transitions in the process of change.

For example, this process of sexuality and gender being considered as examples of the functions of the group becomes particularly important when so-called gender reassignment surgery is being considered in a group setting. Themes of impotence, exclusion, and victimisation are common during such a period, as are anxieties around absent or abusive parents and memories of bodily trauma. These issues, when taken up, can enable the exploration of sensitive areas related to gender and sexuality and broader themes around transition, change, and integration.

> *Jimmy, a trans-man, says he feels cut off and blank. He felt low this week and was not sure why. He resents his body, and it has made him think again about having surgery to alter his body. Julie spoke about her regrets after having a cosmetic facial operation done some years ago to make her face look less Jewish and less like her mother's face. Jimmy stated that he had also found himself doubting having the surgery, which left him feeling confused and ashamed. I picked up on the idea of doubt to say that it might feel hard to speak about the surgery without it feeling like a mistake or an attack on him. In response, Bill recalled a childhood memory of his best friend holding a cross-bow to his head as a joke. Internally, I noted the theme around violence and fear and was aware of wanting to protect them while also continuing the exploration of its meaning. I intervened to note the anxiety as if someone could get hurt. The group became*

quiet for a few minutes. Subsequently, various experiences of trauma of the body emerged, including rape and disability.

There can be difficult exchanges around sexuality and gender in the dialogue of the group that involves enormous pressure to either avoid the topics entirely or solely locate it within the apparently most non-normative individual as if they are to blame. It can be a challenge both for the group analyst and for the group to pursue the ongoing analysis of the conscious and unconscious meanings of gender and sexual identities without fears of intrusion and prejudice, especially given the current public debates on these issues. That fear of prejudice and of being 'politically incorrect' is complicated in terms of what the politics of sexuality and gender in this context might involve. It raises a tension between the psychosocial and the analytic and highlights the institutional political tension within group analysis about how to think about such individuals that tension the individual, medical, and psychoanalytic against the social, group analytic, and discursive. Both modes of thinking are required simultaneously and can easily become destructive and anti-group, to use a further group analytic term, if one or the other takes over entirely in the particular circumstances of the group's themes (Nitsun, 1996). To quote Nitsun:

> *The emphasis on the creative potential of the group . . . is essential. The anti-group is not conceived as a monolithic force that inevitably destroys the group. Rather, it is seen in a complementary relationship with creative group processes but requiring recognition and handling in order that the constructive development of the group can proceed without serious obstruction.*
>
> (Nitsun, 1996:45)

The matrix is a particular group analytic concept that emphasises the role of language and power over language within the whole group. In an analytic group, it is important to hear and accept all voices and that no one voice is the truth, including the group analyst's voice, which I term 'group polyphony'. However unpalatable some voices may be, and however much they may cut across the grain of one's own personal epistemology, it is the difference between 'truths' that enables growth and change by enriching the group's matrix. Group polyphony is a term that attempts to disrupt positions of power and privilege by recognising the equality of voices within the group where the political and apolitical intersect.

A New Speaking-subject of Group Analysis

Recent discussions within the field of group analysis have rightly sought to engage its practice with contemporary political discussions that surround identity. I hesitate with this statement as I prefer to maintain the position that group analytic theory is not a political theory and is instead a theory that aims to de-politicise social dynamics. By stating this, ironically, I run the risk of politicising group analysis into a framework of ideology; to not do so is an impossible task, but it must be frequently checked to remain group analytic. I also recognise that by my writing, I create an unconscious dynamic as a Western white man. I wonder how this chapter might have progressed using a non-Western perspective, for example. I am acutely mindful that there are countries on this planet where being out as gay or trans can result in the death penalty, and I have the privilege to generally write as I wish in the UK.

I do not frame my project within this chapter as if identity is the problem to be solved, but it does come with consequences that can be equally problematic. It is important to reiterate that the movement beyond identity and being 'non-normative' are issues that are not solely located within such members of an analytic group. As mentioned, 'non-normative' sexualities must not be, in group analytic terms, the location of disturbance (Foulkes, 1948; Burman, 2016) or difference (as my preferred term) in an analytic group and, as such, even the category of heterosexuality must be held as equally problematic. However, moving beyond identity means moving towards a shifting, embodied, and fantasised experience of sexuality, erotically and reproductively.

Discussing embodied 'non-normative' sexuality, however, is not an easy task in a group. For example, some Western societies now offer adoption and surrogacy for same-sex couples, and technology is moving rapidly into it being possible for two same-sex gametes to become one fertilised embryo. There has been a rapid expansion of sexualities, genders, and erotic practices. In reality, these future potentialities are not simple options, and some are beyond our everyday technological, discursive, legal, and ethical capabilities. Complex rules of suitability beset adoption that heterosexual reproduction escapes. Such movements within society require a dialogue of bodily sexuality beyond the penis and vagina. However, the potential shame of anal sexuality and the Human Immunodeficiency Virus (HIV) (at least mainly for gay men) provides a heteronormative means to prevent the translation of this movement beyond identity and has maintained same-sex embodied sexuality within an apparent pathology and perversity. These notions of shame, history, reproduction, and eroticism need appropriate space and time in an analytic group if they are to come forward into a conversation and if the group analysands are to move beyond the restrictions of them. The duty to do so, therefore, falls to the group analyst and the training institute.

Group analysis will benefit enormously from an engagement with feminism (including Black feminism) and queer theory, as well as Critical Race Theory. Above all, I hope that group analysts can start to embrace the theory of group analysis without falling too much back upon classical psychoanalysis. That is not to say classical psychoanalysis has no role, for clearly it does. But group analysis also has a robust theoretical voice and can contain multiple discourses within the analytic group, literally and figuratively. The group has to contain and construct its discourse of 'Norm' (Foulkes, 1948) and no-norm within its newly-formed matrix as mobilised by figurations in action. If the matrix is understood to be a kinship network of playful communication and politics between discourses, and if it is mobilised into action by such figurations, then the group has to find a new language with unique symbolic meanings.

Multiple and intersectional desires of others, embodied and contained in an analytic group, become verbalised into language within this polyphony and, consequently, structure the group matrix by it displaying the gaps between discourses. Terms like 'homosexual' and 'trans' will, therefore, have multiple associations and, therefore, begin to fail as terms. By this, I am advocating for a group analytic practice as a way out of reified positionalities and a practice that lets people see the web of unseeable (directly, anyway) power relationships and intersectional identifications and disidentifications that infuse everything. A group analyst, however, must take seriously my caution regarding the location of difference not becoming the location of disturbance. A group must democratically and equally deconstruct such meanings, thereby pushing each member of the group and the group analyst into new and sometimes uncomfortable speaking positions as it finds and problematises locations of difference and similarity. The repetition of these speech acts performs an embodied expansion of the group's knowledge of sexuality and gender. By doing so, a multiplicity of desires becomes creatively bound to the group matrix.

Note

1 This chapter draws upon material published in Anderson, D. (2022) *The Body of the Group: Sexuality and Gender in Group Analysis*. Bicester: Phoenix. It is reproduced with the kind permission of Phoenix Publishing House.

References

Bacha, C. (2005) Commentary on 'Queer Theory' by Katherine Watson. *Group Analysis*, 38(1): 81–85.

Bastian, M. (2006) Haraway's Lost Cyborg and the Possibilties of Transversalism. *Signs: A Journal of Women in Culture and Society*, 43(3): 1027–1049.

Bergler, E. (1947) Differential Diagnosis Between Spurious Homosexuality and Perversion Homosexuality. *Psychiatric Quarterly*, 21(3): 399–409.

Bergler, E. (1948) The Myth of a New National Disease: Homosexuality and the Kinsey Report. *Psychiatric Quarterly*, 22(1): 66–87.

Bergler, E. (1951) *Neurotic Counterfeit Sex*. New York: Grune & Stratton.

Bergler, E. (1956) *Homosexuality: Disease or Way of Life?* New York: Hill & Wang.

Breuer, J. and Freud, S. (1955 [1895]) Studies in Hysteria. In Strachey, J. (ed.) *The Standard Edition of the Complete Psychological Works of Sigmund Freud (SE2)*. London: Hogarth Press [Reprinted 1955].

Burman, E. (2016) The Location of Disturbance: Situating Group Analytic Practice. *CUSP*, 1(2): 1–27.

Elias, N. (1994 [2000]) *The Civilizing Process*. London: Wiley-Blackwells.

Foulkes, S. (1948) *Introduction to Group Analytic Psychotherapy*. London: Karnac.

Haraway, D. (1991) A Cyborg Manifesto: Science, Technology, and Socialist-Feminism in the Late Twentieth Century. In *Simians, Cyborgs and Women: The Reinvention of Nature*. London: Free Association, pp. 149–181.

Lewes, K. (1995) *Psychoanalysis and Male Homosexuality*. Northvale, NJ: Jason Aronson.

Nayak, S. (2014) *Race, Gender and the Activism of Black Feminist Theory: Working with Audre Lorde*. Abingdon: Routledge.

Nitsun, M. (1996) *The Anti-Group*. London: Routledge.

Sedgwick, E. (1990) *Epistemology of the Closet*. Los Angeles: University of California Press.

Stacey, J. (2015) The Unfinished Conversations of Cultural Studies. *Cultural Studies*, 29(1): 43–50.

Watson, K. (2005) Queer Theory. *Group Analysis*, 38(1): 67–81.

Chapter 4

This Is How I Came To Live in Stuckness

Intersectionality, Oppression and 'Affectivism' as a Group Analytic Intervention

Reem Shelhi

Introduction

My first idea for contributing a chapter to this book was to offer a recipe for Libyan Soup. It seemed an apt metaphor for the intersectionality of ingredients that combine, contributing to the flavour of each other while at the same time retaining something of themselves in the meal. Soup also has healing connotations. Rich red Libyan soup, though not well-known, has always been popular with my friends, irrespective of their palate norms and inclinations. As I continued to reflect on this theme, I wondered what was really going on: whether in wanting to be hospitable, I was shrouding my hostility; whether in being playful, I was looking for a way to placate difficult underlying feelings, make my words palatable, easy to swallow. I pondered on the colour red, *seeing red*, wanting to be *properly read*. How do I speak my truth while making sure I don't get stuck in your throat? My own throat is deeply constricted and always has been.

Intersectionality, despite being anti-constricting, does not have a hospitable front. Crenshaw's metaphor of 'traffic' (1998:361) invokes for me neither flow nor congestion but the mangled, cold metallic wreckage of a crash site. This pileup of twisted parts, half, never whole, and yet too much, intimates not only the contours of gender, the skin of ethnicity, the mouth of sexuality and the eyes of shame, but also entangled and intangible clusters, including forms of privilege. The complexity of my contextually kaleidoscopic identity means that themes are so interlinked that one cannot be mentioned without another being inferred and yet another throwing the next off course.

After month upon month of debilitating anxiety and despair, stagnation has given way to movement. Rusty keys are slowly turning the locks of long-abandoned vaults. I'm beginning to see these vaults hold other keys that, though not yet retrieved, will lead me ever more fully back home to myself.

Subjectivity, Timing and Context

The personal nature of this enquiry implies a socio-political dimension that moves it beyond an academic paper to a lived experience of the roots of intersectionality.

DOI: 10.4324/9781003232216-5

It is not my intention to minimize the centrality of childhood in personal develop-ment and trauma, but rather to amplify the equally central and often neglected area of cultural-socio-political oppression and its role in creating and perpetuating disturbance.

Timing and context matters. Vociferous global movements addressing a wide range of oppressive practices attributable to patriarchy, sexism, homophobia, gen-derphobia, ableism and pathologizing are forcing shifts in socio-political and pro-fessional domains that go beyond token inclusion to effortful engagement. The revival of Fanonian literature places decolonization at the centre of humankind's liberation from the wrecking effects of capitalism and the *civilizing process*. The ripples and reverberations of Black Lives Matter have generated renewed and close attention to the question of Palestine, with organizations such as Amnesty Inter-national and Human Rights Watch acknowledging Israel as an 'apartheid state'. In the personal domain, it is no coincidence that my decision to speak out comes in the wake of qualifying as a group analyst who no longer feels constrained by an oftentimes coercive clinical system.

Taking a group analytic setting as a microcosm of the larger cultural-socio-political environment, I draw on post-colonial and Black Feminist literature along with my experience of training as a group analyst, to magnify how differ-ent axes of oppression can interlock, forming sedimented intersectional knots of stuckness and immobility that, if overlooked, ignored or denied, find explosive expression in affects which the social realm condemns as unwelcome distur-bances (Fanon, 2018). I argue that turning away from these affects maintains a climate of socio-intersectional anxiety and alienation, precipitating further dis-turbances and perpetuating cycles of rage and despair. I propose an intervention I term 'Affectivism' as a means of amplifying silenced voices and 'calling out' oppressive situations.

Background

I come from concentric circles of complex overlapping, intertwined and often opposing identities and bio-psycho-socio-cultural systems of power and oppres-sion that are impossible to disentangle. I was born to an English mother who, at an English University, met her Libyan husband, whose family was aligned with the ruling elite. Libya, at this time, was a new Kingdom that had recently gained independence from Italian Colonialism. In the aftermath of World War ll, mixed-race marriages served 'metaphorically as a buttress for a new world order' in which '"love-marriage"' presented 'relationship choice as an inalienable right' and a strengthening of international relations (Piccini, 2021:657). Conversely, there remained on both sides a climate that renounced matrimony between colonizers and colonized subjects, maintaining legitimate concerns about cultural differences. Undeterred, my mother's new life began in the historic city of Tobruk. This idyllic period was shattered by the loss of her husband and eldest child within months of each other. Her marriage to my father, her first husband's youngest brother, saw my arrival a year later. As my mother's youngest and my father's eldest, I am biologically an only child with half-siblings on both sides.

Ghaddafi's 1969 coup d'état-come-revolution brought about a sudden fall from grace. Overnight, my father became a political prisoner, and my family was subject to state surveillance. My siblings were dispersed to boarding schools in Europe, while my mother and I remained stranded in Tripoli. Prevented from leaving, she devised an escape plan across the Libyan-Tunisian border. This audacious and courageous attempt to flee the country when I was six resulted in our betrayal, arrest, imprisonment and a tightened stranglehold of the state's tentacles over our movements. I was a hyperactive and restless child who, despite my mother's enduring efforts, could not be persuaded to read a book. At home, I escaped into music and learnt from her the basic moves of chess. In those moments, it seemed the whole world was neatly organized on a board, and the rules of life were clear.

At the British School in Tripoli, singing hymns inadvertently alerted me to the Arab-Israeli conflict when my mother explained, with a degree of amusement and admiration, the neat circumvention of Zionism when the words to *Noel Noel* were changed from 'born is the King of Israel' to 'born is the King that we all know'. Our delight in this stoically British tuneful act of defiance towards a regime that had incarcerated my father and torn my family apart was tentative. My Christian mother was also an Arabist who studied the language, read extensively on the Middle East and was pro-Palestine. During Islamic holidays, I visited my Libyan aunts, where, with my cousins, we watched the Eid lamb being annually slaughtered. To this day, my own throat intermittently throbs along with intrusive images of it being grated against a giant razor blade, blood gushing out with a sound like deep guttural burping, for words that are snatched away before they can reach my mouth.

My father's much-anticipated release from prison revealed disapproval of my boyish Anglicized persona, which he promptly set about correcting, instructing me to grow my hair and wear dresses, and I was moved me to an Arabic School. His Egyptian education meant that at home, we spoke Arabic with an Egyptian-Libyan dialect. To this day, some Libyans consider us 'foreign'. In fact, on my paternal side, we come from Algeria, Morocco and Chad, and so, like most Libyans, I am part Arab, part African and predominantly Berber. On my maternal side, I am English Anglo-Saxon. And yet, is this not absurd? We all come from stardust and, when cut, bleed the same colour of blood, frantic failing red.

In 1981, against a backdrop of a deteriorating political situation in Libya, I came to England. Despite being in a comparatively more liberal environment, my feelings of displacement heightened. At school, I daydreamed my way through lessons, convinced that if only they could be sung rather than spoken, I would thrive. My teens forced long-standing issues around my sexuality and gender identity to the surface. This, along with a continued sense of isolation and not fitting in, culminated in me dropping out of school without any qualifications. My first encounter with therapy was to be cured of my sexual deviance. My identity as the stupid sibling among my intelligent and well-educated maternal siblings gained traction. The only way I could challenge this was through chess tournaments at home, which I consistently won despite remonstrations that I wasn't playing properly, as prescribed in the books like *real* chess players do. Paradoxically, this ensured that throughout my teens and twenties, my championship status was guarded and fiercely retained, as though my life depended on it.

The AIDS epidemic magnified the demonization of homosexuals, while the introduction of Clause 28 made it illegal to teach about same-sex relationships in schools. Talking about gay sex anywhere seemed taboo. This new social climate confirmed my 'otherness', especially in terms of sexual orientation and non-female conforming identity, adding further to feelings of failure, dislocation and shame. The killing of PC Yvonne Fletcher outside the Libyan Embassy led to the severing of diplomatic relations between Britain and Libya, compounding this sense of dislocation.

The absence of social mirroring is one of the most insidious, inaudibly violent and incrementally corrosive forms of erasure experienced by marginalized people. It is difficult to convey those peculiar feelings of estrangement that come from not having any aspect of one's self-identity reflected in society. Nobody notices, and nobody notices. While growing up, mass media's largely unchallenged depictions of idealized femininity allowed no space for alternative representations of what a woman could be. Wherever I looked, I was reminded of my absence and invisibility. As a living embodiment of unacceptable social norms, attention, when it came, was frequently aggressive, threatening and shame-inducing. In both cultures, the most overt attacks occurred in public spaces; for example, on a train while other passengers pretended nothing was happening, burying their heads in their newspapers. My place of dwelling, then, was a halfway house, and when I ventured outside to walk, it was on a tightrope.

Despite the obstacles I face with reconciling the dominant patriarchal version of Islam with my identity and outlook, I insist on not being estranged from my faith, which I embrace as an existential refrain that transcends the limitations of man-made categorical impositions. Alongside the spiritual and transcendental conduits unfurled through music (Western, Eastern ancient and modern), the celestial wail of Sheikh Al-Minshawi reverently reciting the Qur'an, or the Mu'athin's mournful call to prayer conveys a rhythmic yearning and resignation about coming to terms with being born. Islam means *surrender* to the home that is a foreign land.

Living on the Outside

Chan-Blackburn's observations on the 'discomfort and disappointment of seeing one of your homes suffer due to the actions of the other' (2021) encapsulates a painful dilemma for those of us growing up in worlds pitted against one another. Oftentimes, the double, triple and quadruple binds of injured intersectionality are further exacerbated by the very profession that purports to be about alleviating distress.

And here I have something to confess. As a psychotherapist, it has been difficult to find myself identified with many traits usually ascribed to people with 'disordered' personalities, including living in a paradox that apparently qualifies one as 'borderline' (Cone, 2020:295). And yet, it seems that the nature of our profession attracts many of these 'disordered' types who, feeling compelled by the system to deny their own 'pathology', resort to splitting off these parts and projecting them onto or into others, usually their patients, supervisees or trainees. My point is that many people who cannot make a home in the mainstream find solace in paradox, belonging in the realm of 'stable instability' (Stacey, 2005:193). Within this forced exile, resilient and resourceful strategies emerge. We orbit around ourselves from a distance that paradoxically keeps us connected in ways that don't threaten to split and fragment us into ever tinier pieces. From this outpost, we see the bigger picture clearly. At the same time, perhaps because taken-for-granted truths are not so readily available to us, we insist on the truth wherever we find it. As Cone says, 'a helpful duping of oneself to soften the blow is not available' (2020:295). This mindset that is attuned to paradox exemplifies a tension that results in a need to be 'too sane to be considered crazy and too crazy to be considered sane' (McWilliams, cited in Cone, 2020:296). Feminist theory has a tradition of treating madness as 'a metaphor for female rebellion' (Ahmed, 2017:272) and a 'political act' (Kafai, 2013). The difficulty, however, in disentangling a feminist history from a diagnostic one has come at a cost for women who inhabit 'the mad border body' (Kafai, 2013) and 'expose the instability of the distinction between sanity and madness in how they travel through time and space' (Ahmed, 2017:76).

And yet, the idea of being on the margins of society is not entirely accurate. We have always been inside, at the very heart of oppressive experiences, with 'exceptionally heightened attunement to the expressive landscape' (Koster, 2017:471). The solution, according to Freire, is not to problematize the oppressed nor seek to '"integrate" them into the structure of oppression, but to transform that structure so that they can become "beings for themselves"' (1996:55). This, I think, reflects my identification with the concept of 'coherence' over 'cohesion' in group analysis: I seek reconciliations that reflect the unity of diversity rather than the cohesion of undifferentiated clumped together parts (Ezquerro, 2010; Pines, 1985).

Situating Self in Group Therapy

The group exemplifies a microcosm of its macro socio-political environment in which forms of oppression unfold in a tripartite matrix operating under the sway of a personal and social unconscious (Hopper and Weinberg, 2011). Viewed through an intersectional lens, it is virtually impossible to reduce oppression to one factor.

In this section, I draw upon seven strands of my intersectional identity, which I juxtapose with associated acts of oppression. I locate these in the liminal spaces of a therapeutic group comprizing male and female members who identify as white, heterosexual, privileged professionals: (1) Race, Ethnicity and Culture, (2) Gender, (3) Sexuality, (4) Religion (5) Class, (6) Political Allegiance and (7) Ability. My aim is to illuminate some of the ways in which parallel and multi-directional relationships can intersect to form incrementally interlocking binds of socio-political oppression, external and internalized.

Although these abstracted identity classifications are set out in a linear way, they are inextricably bound up, representing micro, macro and meso nodal points of a system larger than the sum of its parts (Goldstein, 1939; Crenshaw, 1989; Foulkes, 1990; Nayak, 2022).

Race, Ethnicity and Culture (Psychoanalytic Supremacy)

Fanon's observation that 'the majority of Arab territories have been under colonial domination' (2001:171) accounts for the continued uneasy tension between Arabs and the West, which is seen as an 'object of both desire and resentment' (Chen, 2010:217). In this way, the Arab, like the black person, remains a 'fierce critic, as well as both beneficiary and victim, of the project of European modernity' (Burman, 2019:24). As for the West, its historical sense of entitlement to Arab lands, resources and minds has been facilitated by a continued determination to see us as inferior objects of fascination and contempt. The strange eroticization of 'dirty Arabs' (Fanon, 2001:30) situates us as desirable and repellent, barbaric, primitive, irrational and above all, simple people who place their hearts above their heads, as though that is always a bad thing. The history of colonization, the 9/11 attacks, the Iraq war, the war against ISIS, the resurgence of Islamic extremism and, not least, America's alliance with the Zionist state of Israel lends credence to the positioning of Arabs as less than human. Western anti-Arab sentiment is further intensified by feelings of resentment and envy that many harbour towards the oil-rich Arab countries and their inhabitants (Zahrawi, 2020).

'Passing' is associated with efforts by black and mixed-race people to assimilate 'into the dominant white population' (Ababio, 2019:56) and 'Western framework' through the part-internalization of 'colonial objects' (p. 57). It pivots on the notion of privilege, when 'one group has something of value that is denied to the others simply because of the groups they belong to' (Johnson, 2013:17). These descriptions relate to Bhabha's notion of 'mimicry' and the 'not quite white' double-bind of a 'partial presence' in a crowd (2004:122). In approaching mimicry from the standpoint of the colonizer who seeks to tame, refine and incorporate the colonized while also keeping them separate, 'colonial mimicry' conveys 'the desire for a reformed, recognizable Other, as a subject of a difference that is almost the same, but not quite' (Bhabha, 2004:122).

In a colonial environment, being mixed-race exposes the 'crisis of identity' which is 'concealed by the invisibility of the mark of passing' (Ahmed, 1999:97). As a mixed-race woman, embracing the paradox of 'stable instability' frees me to navigate and disrupt the terrain of binary selves fixed in space and time by locating myself 'as the very temporality of passing through and between identity itself without origin or arrival' (Ahmed, 1999:88). However, nestled within this *Hybridization* (p. 97) is a catch; the 'radical and transgressive practice' that aims to dislocate and destabilize the systems of knowledge upon which identity and subjectivity are predicated and 'precariously rests' (p. 88) overlooks 'the means by which relations of power are secured, paradoxically, through this very process of destabilization' (p. 89).

In exploring the relationship between psychoanalysis and race, Blechner acknowledges that 'racist and other prejudices' are 'silently, perhaps unconsciously, imprinted on its theories and practices' (2020:252). The conductor of groups comprizing minoritized individuals should guard against the slide into conflating a framework of inherent asymmetry with psychoanalytic supremacy, a stance and attitude that intentionally confuses having a particular kind of knowledge with condescending certainty. For example, being emphatically told that one is 'using race' to 'avoid addressing more personal issues' exemplifies the dangerous and especially insidious psychic violence and foreclosure enacted by the analyst who has 'the power to name the psychology of another' (Sheehi and Sheehi, 2022:62).

Having a valency for other people's projections, wishes and fantasies can become amplified with intersectional identities. Perhaps because we confound the need to sort, label and categorize, the fine line we tread exposes us to falling between the cracks of other people's missing parts; our ambiguity can make us a mutable canvas for other's projections, becoming whatever suits them in their context. My own need for belonging, if only at the level of *meaning-making,* results in my collusion with this dynamic, thus going from being different to being 'differently situated' in different contexts (Crenshaw, 1991:1250). Arabs, after all, if nothing else, are a hospitable people.

Gender (Misogynoir)

Crenshaw's seminal paper on minoritized women shows how institutional expectations based on 'inappropriate non-intersectional contexts' coupled with the 'effects of multiple subordination' adds insult into deeply ingrained injuries, ultimately thwarting any 'opportunity for meaningful intervention on their behalf' (1991:1251). Indeed, 'Intersectional subordination' (1991:1249) conveys the intersectional racialized position of women not only in relation to group therapy but also training institutions. Women are often expected to absorb and 'laugh off' sexist remarks, but I sometimes wondered, as a mixed-race Arab trainee in a group setting, whether this developed into direct misogynistic aggressions or insults such as being told, 'shut your mouth'. Whilst trainee group therapists can bring concerns to the institution of training management, the response of 'take it back to the group' is tricky when the therapy group itself is the problem. In addition, refusal can be characterized as a 'resistant trainee'.

'Misogynoir' is a term that describes the interlocking of racism and sexism (Bailey, 2021:1) along with homophobia and prescriptive expressions of gender (Bailey and Trudy, 2018) that women from black or minority groups experience. Originally, in the context of digital media, it was extended to include 'social or institutional environments' (Trudy, cited in Kwarteng et al., 2022:165). Nayak's paper on 'racialized misogyny' links 'splitting and part-object relationships' with fractured, cut-up, fetishized identities of Asian and black women along with queer, non-binary or gay women who 'do not fit dominant white, heteronormative able-bodied constructions'. (2021:523). Underscoring the importance of 'projective identification, countertransference and resonance' in enabling 'a naming of the nameless dread of racialized misogyny' (p. 523), Nayak offers ways of 'disrupting essentialist constructs of gender and sexuality' (p. 522).

Bourdieu's 'the pertinence principle' refers to a discriminating filter that selects and 'defines all the characteristics of persons or things which can be perceived, and perceived as positively or negatively interesting' (2010:477). The hallmark of this filter is its capacity to 'demand that certain things are brought together, and others kept apart' (Bourdieu, 2010:476–477). The pertinence principle is also bound up with toxic masculinity. My identity and appearance as a non-conforming strong woman often result in my being misgendered. However, in situations where my gender is known, my appearance has been perceived as a threat to masculinity, dealt with by identifying me with masculine traits rather than affirming my gender as a woman who doesn't conform to stereotypes. This 'dis-gendering' negates my sense of self as a woman, leaving only the binary position of male available as a means of relating to me. The implication is that if I want to 'be one of the boys' (I don't), then I should 'take it like a man'. Despite increasing literature challenging the 'angry black woman' trope, women's anger, particularly minoritized women, remains unwelcome (Kent, 2021). Silencing practices such as 'tone-management', which is 'aimed at directly managing subordinate groups' *angry knowledge*' (Bailey, 2018:97 – my italics), tend to surface. Stoute's paper, 'Black Rage' (2021), links fury to 'moral injury'. Here, indignation 'mobilised for the purposes of defence or psychic growth' is understood as a 'compromise formation that is a functional adaptation for oppressed people' who suffer various forms of 'trauma' and 'degradation' (2021:259).

Sexuality (Homophobia)

Stigma describes 'the situation' of individuals who are 'disqualified from full social acceptance' (Goffman, 1990:9) while being 'continuously available for perception' (p. 124). While there have been marked improvements in society's attitudes to same-sex sexuality, exposure to 'sexual stigma', a 'stereotype consisting of negative judgements based on heteronormative attitudes', persists (Ingoglia et al., 2020:137). This external factor becomes internalized by members of a sexual minority resulting in 'a self-directed negative attitude', including 'internalised homophobia, internalised homonegativity, or internalised heterosexism' (p. 138).

The societal tendency to make links between sexual orientation and trauma is a politically sensitive minefield (Roberts et al., 2013), but one which also endures. It is a dilemma that I have grappled with most of my life, only recently coming to understand its harmful moral and ethical implications. In fact, it is only recently that I have come to regard the faulting of sexuality as nothing less than a direct assault on the most private, intimate and vulnerable realm of the human psyche; a violation and intrusion that induces unimaginable forms of suffering on those of us who undergo this experience.

The idea of trauma/fault in the context of sexuality often pits the demand for repair against impossibility, establishing a cycle of despair, a trap. Under conditions of such oppression, the oppressed hold on to the belief that their sexuality can be 'fixed', that it is only a matter of time and the cure will come. Until then, the present is frozen; we cannot move on. The hope for redemption and deliverance is always in the future, *mañana, tomorrow, inshallah,* always postponed. Meanwhile, for the oppressor, life goes on as normal, supposing that only by working through trauma can the oppressed fully join them in their socially accepted world. If one's deviant sexuality has not been repaired, then not enough hard work has been done: 'Dig deeper', something has been buried down below. We must drag it up, even if, in doing so, our very core, the essence of who we have become, must be dismantled, undone, fragmented further. This exploitation of our 'fundamental need to relate' (Foulkes, 1964:109) induces perpetual feelings of shame, defined by De Young as the 'experience of one's felt sense of self disintegrating in relation to a dysregulating other' (2015:18). This is how we come to live in stuckness, perpetual disintegration, always reaching for that impossible and ridiculous goal, interpersonally and intrapersonally, to be made 'normal' again.

In a group context, a question linking being gay to trauma may be immediately validated rather than held and thought about, overshadowed by a seemingly endorsed belief that if trauma could be worked through and overcome, gay people would be 'normalised'. Attempts to 'cure' undermines the mutability of sexual relationships by linking mutability to 'possibility for change' instead of 'psycho-bio-socially and contextually' driven choices that do not have to be standardized or regulated. Over time, we can see once again the same pattern, a toxic attitude and approach which causes minoritized subjects 'to doubt their ability to make judgements about their moral worth' (Bailey, 2018:94–95).

Religion (Islamophobia and Rationalization)

A detailed study of media depictions of Muslims in the UK revealed considerable problems. The most prevalent was the association of Islam with violence and, by extension, Muslims having a 'a unique penchant for it' (Hamid, 2021:64). People with Muslim and/or Arabic names are likely to experience far greater rejection when gaining employment (Milsom, 2021) and face greater housing discrimination (Murchie and Pang, 2018; Carlsson and Eriksson, 2014). An accepted way of dealing with this problem in large swathes of the Arab Muslim population is to Westernize their names as a means of 'passing', leading ultimately to self-alienation and, I contend, increased self-loathing.

The conflation between Islam and terrorism leads to unconscious bias (Bayoumi, 2018). Revealing one's faith can evoke feelings of anxiety, leading to a propensity to 'explain oneself' as a way of reassuring others. On the other hand, being Muslim can carry an increased willingness not to discuss one's faith or to 'silence ourselves to allay fears of surveillance' (Ghalaini, 2020:99). These coping mechanisms can promote internalized Islamophobia instead of changing the social outlook. Anti-islamophobia efforts, while mostly laudable and effective, can risk 'tokenizing' Muslims who are then expected to feel indebted for being included.

But there is something else. The oppositional relationship between psychoanalysis and religion in which the former's primary pursuit of 'justification of the subjective experience' (Besner, 2009:85) can lead to a disavowal of the latter. Religion, wrote Freud, is a 'universal obsessional neurosis' comparable to 'the neurosis of children' (Freud, 1927:43). A Muslim may conceal or downplay religious sensibilities that risk being perceived as childish or irrational. The desire to gain the dominant group's acceptance may result in identifying with ridicule or conferring with the assumption that 'to suppose that what science cannot give us we can get elsewhere' is tantamount to self-deception (Freud, 1927:56). This has subtle and pertinent connections to Nayak's observations on the fetishization of rationality and its function in psychoanalysis as one of the 'mechanisms of regulation and control' (2019:358).

Class (Splitting)

Collins (1998) reminds us of the importance of acknowledging areas of privilege in intersectionality since these will also have an effect, although it may be hard to fit into neat explanations.

Accent, dialect and vocabulary are indicators of class and power structures. Baratta argues that 'accents are often merely a proxy for the judgements we make of their speakers' (2018:62), while Shuck contends 'speakers perform ideologies' (2004:199). The latter's study of the dogma of language or 'Ideology of Nativeness' (Shuck 2004:196) reveals how ideological performances follow binary 'formulaic discourse patterns' (Subtirelu, 2015:37) that situate the other as 'foreign, incomprehensible, and even frightening' (Shuck, 2004:196). For example, complaints such as 'couldn't understand a word they were saying', although ostensibly signalling the desire for communication, reveal two things: An 'Us/Them' split and a connection to 'broader issues of political power and social exclusion through their intersection with other oppressive ideologies, such as racism' (Subtirelu, 2015:36; Shuck, 2004).

English accents continue to function as expressions and indicators of a person's class and, by extension, their wealth and social standing (Manstead, 2018). Received Pronunciation (RP) has been historically associated with being 'highly educated and intelligent' (Baratta, 2018:62). The notion of 'received pronunciation', however, also functions as a means of division and control (Bourdieu, 1991; Mugglestone, 2003). Where does my accent place me? My relationship with English has been fraught with privileges and contradictions, confusing the boundaries between authentic modes of being and performativity. The English I learned from my mother was inflected with British upper middle-class intonations. Yet there is also something else distantly in the background, which is hard to place and ambiguous. My education, while short-lived, was in private institutions. At the same time, my accent carries authority and gives me license to step forward and announce myself without apology. Ultimately, however, my accent functions as my sword and shield on both sides of the colonial/colonized divide, capable of both legitimizing and denouncing me. Context is everything.

Political Allegiances (Pinkwashing)

Blechner, recognizing the continued Jewish influence on psychoanalysis, points out that while much attention has been given to anti-semitism in the literature, other forms of racism and oppression have been largely neglected (2020). A theme that I downplayed in group therapy was my political identity as an Arab-Muslim among predominately heterosexual, Jewish and white intellectuals (Stobo, 2011; Salm, 2012).

Sheehi and Sheehi's ground-breaking book *Psychoanalysis Under Occupation* (2022) offers an uncompromising depiction of the many deeply disguised forms of clinical violence, conscious and/or unconscious – lurking in asymmetrical colonizer-colonized/oppressor-oppressed motifs. For an Arab, joining a predominately privileged white Jewish-led group may feel precarious and induce feelings of ambivalence. At the same time, the need for validation can override gut feelings. In my experience, joining an analytic group felt like joining the inner chamber, the intellectual heavyweights. Fanon's observations on the subservient toxic gratitude born out of the 'master who allowed his slaves to eat at his table' (Fanon, 1952:194), intersecting with that part of my Arab identity that wanted to be accepted by the Jewish elite (Srour, 2015) may elucidate this psychic quagmire.

In this setting, my resentment of Israel and its treatment of Palestinians was matched by an unwanted sense of inferiority and guilt for seeking out the knowledge of the 'Jewish science' (Sheehi and Sheehi, 2022:16). In my experience, exploration of the Holocaust and anti-semitism is often at the expense of the atrocities being inflicted on the Palestinian people. Shame, Arab shame from feeling inferior (Srour, 2015), and Jewish-Israeli shame from knowing only too well the monstrosities Israel is visiting upon Palestinians may account for this disavowal (Shoshani, Shoshani and Shinar, 2010). Israel's ethnic cleansing of the Palestinians, along with Islamophobia, are factors that, though written about, continue to be neglected in practice. Furthermore, Jewish practitioners continue to underestimate the impact of the Israeli occupation of Palestine on Arabs and Muslims all over the world. An Arab-Muslim experiencing group therapy in a Jewish household setting can bring conflictual feelings to the surface. There is a climate of fear and anxiety in talking about Palestine, marked primarily by the way that anti-semitism is used at every turn to silence thinking.

Pinkwashing is a relatively recent term coined to describe the deliberate exploitation and amplification of pro-LGBTQ+ rights – evidence of liberalism and democracy – as a means of obfuscating and legitimizing other abuses (Anderson, 2019). It is essentially a splitting technique, a 'demean, divide and rule' strategy deployed to maintain minority subjugation (Blackmer, 2019). Pro-Palestinian women who identify as Muslim and gay may face attempts at silencing by having those different aspects of themselves set against each other. For example, the retort 'at least in Israel you can hold your girlfriend's hand in public' is used to excuse or distract from atrocities against Palestinians.

Ability ('Disorder' Pathologies)

The dominance of a medical model is being challenged by advocating a shift from a pathology paradigm to a neurodiversity paradigm (Walker, 2021; de Houting, 2019; Glassgold, 2022).

Borderline Personality Disorder (BPD) is a deeply painful and 'highly prevalent' condition (Luyton et al., 2019:88) underpinned by paradoxes and double binds (Stanghellini and Rosfort, 2013). People with borderline organizations are considered 'fragile and aggressive patients' (Ruggiero, 2012:93) who are 'notoriously difficult to treat' (Levy et al., 2006:483). Indeed, it is not uncommon, inside and outside the mental health profession, to hear references to 'borderlines' in disparaging tones. Borderlines often cope with stigmatization by identifying with it. The borderline's self-stigmatization, which arises 'from one's acceptance of societal prejudices' is a 'maladaptive process' (Grambal et al., 2016:2439) comparable to malignant identifications and internalized oppression. In groups, accusations such as 'you've lost your thinking capacity' or that one is 'incapable of using the group' can be experienced as undermining and destabilizing the capacity to think (Bion, 1967) in a way that is particularly diminishing for people who are neurodiverse. Its persistence over time leads to an incremental grinding down of any sense of self, culminating in what has been powerfully summed up as 'the loss of the right to appear' (Woloshyn and Savage, 2020:2).

Recently, the anti-pathologizing term 'neuroqueer' has emerged to counter the bio-medical model as 'the practice of queering (subverting, defying, disrupting, liberating oneself from) neuronormativity and heteronormativity simultaneously' (Walker, 2021:113–114).

Projective identification has been described as an 'all-consuming' phenomenon that can 'erode one's sense of worth as a human being' (Messina, 2019:106). It originated with Klein's theory of a 'felt to be the "bad" self' entering 'the mother's body' and taking 'control of it' (Klein, 1952:69). This process of infiltrating and taking over corresponds to processes of colonization (Fanon, 2001, 2018). Projective identification is also a process ascribed to borderline organizations. What is notable, however, is that it is always implicated in the context of the 'hateful, destructive feelings the patient violently plunges into the therapist' (Gans, 2018:5), not the other way around. The tendency to focus on projective identification as originating in the 'patient' can be seen as another way of maintaining psychoanalytic supremacy. Addressing this imbalance entails establishing methods of considering this phenomenon in bi-directional, even multidirectional ways.

Mental Hygiene

In clinical work, whatever our position, reflexivity and self-accountability are important. However, in processes of decolonization, reflecting on the nuances of unconscious processes often becomes a luxury that many can ill-afford. In the context of abusive (not unequal) power relations, people who have been marginalized are demanding that certain conditions be met before going back to the business of reflecting upon the very real and important unconscious processes that affect us all and implicate us all in acts of oppression.

Oppressive conduct couched in clinical interventions is easy to detect by the receiver but often difficult to substantiate, particularly when oppressions intersect and overlap, making distinctions between them seem impossible. As clinicians, this places us in positions of responsibility while accentuating the importance of honesty and integrity in our conduct. Foulkes's own awareness of the power invested in conductors and the importance of not abusing it is implicit in his observation that a conductor's 'personality and method are the most important individual factors' influencing the group (Foulkes, 1975b:3). When the inherently asymmetrical positions that characterize psychoanalytic spaces are further complicated by intersectional forms of dominance and oppression, the term 'mental hygiene' (Foulkes, 1964:179, 1975b:154), though not defined in Foulkes writing, stands out as an important term to describe the 'right attitude in the therapist or the main conditions of the successful handing of a group' (1964:201).

Recognizing that conductors' technique arises from their attitude (Foulkes, 1964:50), I suggest that 'mental hygiene' be anchored as a group analytic 'maxim' (Foulkes, 1975b:153) that incorporates the conductor's own 'principles of conduct' (p. 87). This begins with recognizing their role as 'the first servant of the group' (Foulkes, 1975b:107), an anti-colonial stance espousing humility, the courage to look within, face one's own shortcomings and respond with integrity and accountability to mistakes and/or injuries. Foulkes further advocates a 'non-manipulative' (1975b:133) attitude, without any agenda to 'use the group' to fulfil narcissistic wishes (Foulkes, 1948:139). He insists that we know and stay aware of our 'enormous suggestive influence' (Foulkes, 1975a:268) and for the conductor not to pose 'as a shining example or as an all-knowing physician who can cure his patients' (1948:142). The conductor's aim always being to exemplify a 'modesty' which comes from 'self-confidence' (Foulkes, 1964:65) to practice and promote 'tolerance . . . independence . . . and an open mind of new experiences' (Foulkes, 1964:57).

Leaving the Group

Fanon has used the term 'dialectical substitution' (2018 [1952]:129) to describe a discombobulating process of inverted code-switching which increases confusion and self-doubt so that effectively, as Fanon notes, 'they were countering my irrationality with rationality, my rationality with their "true rationality." I couldn't hope to win' (2018 [1952]:111).

An incrementally corrosive atmosphere of an 'exclusionary matrix' (Weegman, 2014:104) will start to take its toll. As Wilderson observes, 'there is a struggle to maintain one's sanity in a context in which your consciousness is at war with the given' (Hartman and Wilderson, 2003:196). Experiences of being gaslighted can lead to feelings of going mad. A caustic group culture can steadily disintegrate into a cesspit of rivalrous and sadomasochistic exchanges and malignant mirroring (Zinkin, 1992), setting up an environment ripe for scapegoating (Kent, 2021).

The group analytic concept of *condensation* posits that a symptom, instead of being caused by 'a single event', arises 'out of multiple traumas, frequently analogous and repeated' (Fanon, 2018:123). Zahrawi reminds us,

A person's identity is not an assemblage of separate affiliations, nor a kind of loose patchwork: it is like a pattern drawn on a tightly stretched parchment. Touch just one part of it, just one allegiance, and the whole person will react, the whole drum will sound.

(2020:124)

The problem, Sheehy and Nayak contend, 'is not a matter of how your message is transmitted' but rather 'refusal of the message' itself (2020:239). My counter-refusal in my group to yield to pressure and be brought into line or 'be managed' meant something had to give. I left the group.

Aftermath

As a result of my own experiences, I have long pondered the question, how is it that people can harbour strong feelings about abuses of power yet not speak out? What is it that makes people choose to turn away from moral injuries? What are the inhibiting factors? The conception of the human being as a 'particle of a group' (Foulkes and Anthony, 1957:234) or a nodal point in a network implies not only that we are connected but also each other's consequences are connected. Foulkes remarked that the moral and ethical responsibilities implied in this can lead us to turn a blind eye to outbreaks of social disturbance (1990:225), causing the 'bystander effect'. Contributory factors may include theoretical frameworks that rely on paternalistic individualistic psychoanalytic interpretations that do not adequately account for complex social dynamics. An example is an emphasis on the idea of the 'social unconscious' at the expense of 'social consciousness'. In this way, the social is *disturbingly unconscious* in group analysis. Finally, even when social or 'critical consciousness' emerges (Freire, 1996), people are afraid to act on what they know. Paradoxically, this can be attributed in a significant part to Foulkes's 'Basic Law' and its push for sameness and conformity (Foulkes, 1948:29). Trainees, in particular face a dilemma, on the one hand, being encouraged to talk as freely as possible about their thoughts, feelings and experiences, while at the same time being kept under a sort of *super-egoic panopticon gaze* that impedes authentic engagement and, ironically, stifles professional development. The result is disingenuous group therapies where many choose to avoid attention and get through their training rather than immerse themselves wholeheartedly in the business of being human.

Affectivism

Group Analysis is a radical, personal and socio-political enterprise underpinned by 'an open-ended list of ethical and political values' (Benjamin and Tucker, 2021:8). Turning away from or pathologizing socio-political disturbances exacerbates a climate of raging despair, leading to further 'explosions' and increasing alienation. What is the answer? In *The Wretched of the Earth*, Fanon concedes 'decolonisation is always a violent phenomenon' (2001:27). Furthermore, violence escalates when oppressive 'attitudes do not change' (Lorde, 2019:123). Hence, in the context of decolonization, the regulation of affect as a component of our work raises some challenging moral imperatives around the importance of guarding against the exploitation of this regulating tendency, which, I contend, paradoxically becomes a sort of weaponization of safety.

De Beauvoir reminds us that 'the oppressor would not be so strong if he did not have accomplices among the oppressed themselves' (1948:98). My concept of *Affectivism* relates to this. It comes from having encountered, throughout my life and significantly during my training as a group analyst, situations where I became the location of disturbance for expressing opinions that weren't sanctioned by the mainstream. When, behind the scenes, people expressed quiet solidarity, I often wanted to say, 'Why didn't you speak up then?'

Our awareness that the (un)conscious communication of one person is often heard more clearly by another who stands outside has strong psycho-social and moral implications. Are we not then each other's ears? And if so, are we not also each other's eyes? And if so, each other's guardians, voices? Each other's affect? Shay's definition of moral injury is specific and wide. It is a 'betrayal of what's right . . . by someone who holds legitimate authority . . . in a high stakes situation' (2014:183). The criteria of these three elements can be interpreted differently by different people, so while I draw on this definition, my focus is on injuries that arise more generally and in wider contexts.

'Affectivism' (which combines *affect* with *activism*) is proposed as a multifaceted, destabilizing, decolonizing and de-pathologizing concept and group analytic intervention that exemplifies turning to and moving towards (rather than turning away from) the intuitively felt sense of emotional, psychological or material consequence of oppression. Affectivism invokes the Fanonian clinician who can help to revive and promote 'subjective agentic capacities', these being not only capacities to 'reflect', but also 'to act'. (Burman, 2020:10). It can intervene at any stage in the trajectory of affective intensities, from faint and subtle feelings of unease to outright indignation, sadness and despair. I am proposing it initially in the context of moral injuries, although it has wider applications that cannot be discussed here.

Affectivism aims to transform locations of disturbance into *locations of discovery*, espousing a *curious rather than curative* approach. In difficult and precarious situations, it asks us to do a double take, to think again about what just happened, within ourselves and in relation to others. As such, it is aligned with *expressive rather than repressive* interventions and with *coherence* rather than *cohesion* so that even the most violent or threatening forms of affect can be given room to breathe, if not to vent. This is not an argument for wild, free-flowing rage. However, taking seriously the idea that the anger of the oppressed 'is loaded with information and energy' (Lorde, 2019:121), it is an invitation, particularly to us group analysts, to step up to the plate and involve ourselves more courageously in addressing moral injuries on both personal and socio-political levels. We need to develop more resilience in facilitating the expression and toleration of affects, including anger, hurt and grief, recognizing this as vital to decolonization and transformational work. Affectivism can be a way of diluting overwhelming feelings, an offer to share the load, exemplifying the difference between holding it together and holding it, together.

Affectivism is bound up with all affects (emotions and feelings) that are rooted in silencing and/or oppressive injuries. The peeled-back nature of affect speaks to the Fanonian invitation, 'Why not simply try to touch the other, feel the other, discover each other?' (Fanon, 2018 [1952]:206). What would it be like to enquire, how are you? What just happened there? What's going on? Is there something that one of us missed? This would enable a paradigm shift from the question 'What's wrong with you?' to 'What's happened to you?' (Helbich and Jabr, 2022:314)

People who have internalized forms of oppression are in a double double-bind stemming from, on the one hand the desire to be free but also a terror of that freedom (Freire, 1996). The master-slave dynamic ensures that colonized minds are simultaneously locked into an existential vacuum and locked out of participating in the everyday living familiar to more integrated people (Fanon, 2018). Through 'recognising as social and systemic what was formerly perceived as isolated and individual' (Crenshaw, 1991:1241–1242), affectivisim may contribute to initiating 'an agentic voluntarism that is forged through the social, rather than abstracted from it' (Burman, 2019:24). Energy, for better or for worse, can make things happen. Affectivisim asks us to be attuned to the energies arising within ourselves and those around us, to notice and name encounters with injustice, those *felt-sense split-second moments* of someone's dignity being compromised or their integrity violated. Naming something is in itself an intervention. Affectivism goes further by anchoring naming into 'muscle memory'. Moreover, when people have the idea that they have the power to intervene, it makes them more likely to act.

Affectivism has a socio-political dimension. It bridges the gap between the clinic and the wider socio-political arena, reflecting the idea that the personal is political and linking this overtly to the group analyst. It is solidarity-in-action. It also takes seriously the notion of 'socio-political grief', a term implying the deep collective and/or personal loss and despair experienced by individuals because of governmental or institutional policies, ideologies, and practices (Bordere and Harris, 2022). In this context, we might surmise that it is not only 'the *shadow* of the *object'* which *'fell upon* the ego' (Freud, 1917:249) but the shadow of the system which fell upon the subject. Affectivism is also anti-pathology, highlighting that while it might feel dangerous to look, it can be more dangerous to look away. Here, affectivism offers a way of harnessing and channelling that 'well-stocked arsenal of anger potentially useful against those oppressions' whether personal, institutional or in the wider socio-political arena 'which brought that anger into being' (Lorde, 2019:141).

Oppression thrives on splitting, fragmentation, division, disconnection and categorization (Nayak, 2022). I have found that even scholars who are proficient in theorizing about oppressive practices and the means of overcoming them struggle to implement their own ideas. As Nayak explains, oppression's very target is unity and multiplicity, systems big and small that are coherent and interdependent and which become the target of attempts to 'keep separating the inseparable' (Gunnarsson, cited in Nayak, 2022:325). This is a key reason why Black Feminist theory insists on the indivisibility and inseparability of theory and practice. Lorde reminds us: 'The master's tools will never dismantle the master's house' (Lorde, 2019:105). In a similar vein, Helbich and Jabr offer three key actions for resisting the internalization of oppression in any context: First, challenging the concept of neutrality. In this ethical approach of '"non-neutrality"', suffering is explored in terms of 'the conditions that create it' (2022:306), including the effects of 'political violence' (p. 307). Secondly, 'directing feelings outward, to those who oppress, instead of inward' (p. 311), and thirdly, prioritizing a collective human rights framework over an individual trauma framework (Helbich and Jabr, 2022). The relocation of trauma to the collective realm corresponds to the notion of 'sibling authority' and 'being of alongside' (Parker, 2020:78), facilitating solidarity and 'community resilience' (Sousa et al., 2013:242).

It is important to stress that affectivism does not, in the first instance, rely on cognition but asks us to be attuned to our feelings and inner *felt sense of something*. We know that centuries of oppression have made women 'come to distrust that power which rises from our deepest and non-rational knowledge' (Lorde, 2019:43). Affectivism mobilizes affective and intuitive faculties in and of themselves. There are truths and forms of knowledge imbedded in those affects that arise before we've even had a chance to fully comprehend them. When these surface, we feel/know we are a witness to something, yet we often turn away rather than recognize and respond to what is happening.

Conclusion

The points of intersection between external (micro)aggressions and one's own internalized self-hate are the most insidious and dangerous. Here lie the cracks and incisions into which the disease of oppression trickles, snaking its way through our bloodstream and into the inner most chamber, our hearts: that symbolic keeper not of logic, but of our feelings. But inside this numinous cauldron, invisible fires of intuition still rage, every so often spitting flames and shooting sparks so high that they evade capture. In *The Famished Road*, Ben Okri writes, 'This is what you must be like. Grow wherever life puts you down' (2016:46).

We can avoid the pitfalls of getting sucked into the mainstream, neither conforming to the noxious elements of a white Western patriarchal paradigm nor those of other oppressive cultures. Standing 'outside from within' these systems will not be easy. The key is finding one's tribe, a group of like-minded and similarly experienced people who recognize and resonate with our loneliness and longing, along with our relentless capacity for hope and resilience. At the same time, we should continue questioning our own assumptions. We like to think we know ourselves, particularly in our line of work, that we are self-aware and that it is the other who has changes to make. But in what kind of way and according to whose ideology? In the final analysis, getting in touch with our own internalized oppressors is 'the true focus of revolutionary changes' (Lorde, 2019:117). We are, after all, each other's mirrors.

I will conclude by returning to the metaphor of traffic and its wreckage of tongue-tied traumas. When we encounter a traffic jam, our first instinct is to look for an escape route. Sitting in the sticky heat of stuckness is hard to tolerate. Intersectionality, I realize, asks us to do precisely this: not to turn away from ourselves.

Finding my way into this paper has been arduous, sometimes retraumatizing, and could not have been achieved without the patience, understanding and support of colleagues. As I have stayed with the process, those mangled lumps of twisted metal are starting to melt, and the full force of my oppression is dawning. Painful as this has been, it has also provided pointers for escape and liberation. I insist on my belonging, and while my difference has come at a heavy price, it is one that I do not regret paying. My work continues, unpicking the knots of injured intersectionality one stitch at a time and learning to stand – upright and embodied – in my own power.

References

Ababio, B. (2019) Not Yet at Home, An Exploration of Aural and Verbal Passing Among African Migrants in Britain. In Ababio, B. and Littlewood, R. (eds.) *Intercultural Therapy, Challenges, Insights and Developments*. London and New York: Routledge, Taylor and Francis Group.

Ahmed, S. (1999) Passing Through Hybridity. *Theory, Culture & Society*, 16(2): 87–106.

Ahmed, S. (2017) *Living a Feminist Life*. Durham, NC: Duke University Press.

Anderson, J. (2019) Pinkwashing. In Chiang, H. (ed.) *Global Encyclopedia of Lesbian, Gay, Bisexual, Transgender, and Queer ILGBTQ) History*. New York: Charles Scribner's Sons.

Bailey A. (2018) On Anger, Silence, and Epistemic Injustice. Royal Institute of Philosophy Supplement, 84: 93–115.

Bailey, M. (2021) *Misogynoir Transformed, Black Women's Digital Resistance*. New York: New York University Press.

Bailey, M. and Trudy (2018) On Misogynoir: Citation, Erasure, and Plagiarism. *Feminist Media Studies*, 18(4): 762–768. https://doi.org/10.1080/14680777.2018.1447395

Baratta, A. (2018) Index. In *Accent and Teacher Identity in Britain: Linguistic Favouritism and Imposed Identities*. London: Bloomsbury Academic, pp. 209–210. Bloomsbury Collections [Accessed online 28th February 2023].

Bayoumi, M. (2018) How Does It Feel to Be a Problem? *Amerasia Journal*, 27(3): 69–77.

Benjamin, A. and Tucker, S. (2021) We've All Got Skin the Game: National Diversity Working Group: Power, Privilege and Position. *Group Analysis*, 54(3): 437–459.

Besner, R. (2009) Self or No Self: Psychoanalytic and Buddhist Perspectives on Neuroendocrine Events and Subjective Experience. In *Taboo or Not Taboo*. London: Karnac Books Limited.

Bhabha, H. (2004 [1994]). *The Location of Culture*. London: Routledge Classics, Taylor & Francis Group.

Bion, W. R. (1967) Attacks on Linking. In *Second Thoughts: Selected Papers on Psychoanalysis*. London: Karnac.

Blackmer, C. (2019) Pinkwashing. *Israel Studies*, 24(2).

Blechner, M. (2020) Racism and Psychoanalysis: How They Affect One Another. *Contemporary Psychoanalysis*, 56(2–3): 245–254.

Bordere, T. and Harris, D. (2022) *A Q&A with Drs. Tashel Bordere and Darcy Harris, the Co-Presenters of Our First 2022 Workshop – Sociopolitical Grief (January 21st)*. www.portlandinstitute.org/sociopolitical-grief

Bourdieu, P. (1991) *Language and Symbolic Power*. Trans. G. Raymond and M. Adamson. Cambridge: Polity Press.

Bourdieu, P. (2010 [1984]) *Distinction, A Social Critique of the Judgement of Taste* (Routledge Classics). London: Taylor and Francis Group.

Burman, E. (2019) *Fanon, Education, Action: Child as Method*. Oxford: Routledge.

Burman, E. (2020) Frantz Fanon and Revolutionary Group Praxis. *Group Analysis*, 54(2): 169–188.

Carlsson, M. and Eriksson, S. (2014) Discrimination in the Rental Market for Apartments. *Journal of Housing Economics*, 23: 41–54. https://doi.org/10.1016/j.jhe.2013.11.004 [Accessed online 28th February 2023].

Chan-Blackburn, G. (2021) Writing about Simryn Gill's Photographs. *Tate Magazine*, Summer Edition.

Chen, K. H. (2010) *Asia as Method: Toward Deimperialization*. Chapel Hill, NC: Duke University Press.

Collins, P. H. (1998) The Tie that Binds: Race, Gender and US Violence. *Ethnic and Racial Studies*, 21(5): 917–938.

Cone, D. (2020) Double-Think, Double-Binds and the Secret History of the Borderline Personality Disorder. *British Journal of Psychotherapy*, 36(2): 294–302.

Crenshaw, K (1989) Demarginalizing the Intersections of Race and Sex: A Black Feminist Critique of Antidiscrimination Doctrine, Feminist Theory and Antiracist Politics. *University of Chicago Legal Forum*, 1989(1), Article 8.

Crenshaw, K. (1991) Mapping the Margins: Intersectionality, Identity Politics, and Violence Against Women of Colour. *Stanford Law Review*, 43(6): 1241–1300.

Crenshaw, K. (1998) A Black Feminist Critique of Antidiscrimination Law and Politics. In Kairys, D. (ed.) *The Politics of Law: A Progressive Critique*, 3rd ed. New York: Basic Books, pp. 356–379.

de Beauvoir, S. (1948) *The Ethics of Ambiguity*. Trans. from the French by B. Frechtman. New York: Philosophical Library.

den Houting, J. (2019) Neurodiversity: An Insider's Perspective. *Autism*, 23(2): 271–273. https://doi.org/10.1177/1362361318820762

De Young, P. (2015) *Understanding and Treating Chronic Shame: A Relational/Neurobiological Approach*. London: Routledge.

Ezquerro, A. (2010) Cohesion and Coherency in Group Analysis. *Group Analysis*, 43(4): 496–504.

Fanon, F. (2001 [1961]) *The Wretched of the Earth*. Trans. C. Farrington. London: Penguin Modern Classics.

Fanon, F. (2018 [1952]) *Black Skin, White Masks*. Trans. from the French by R. Philcox. New York: Grove Press.

Foulkes, S. H. (1948) *Introduction to Group Analytic Psychotherapy*. London: Karnac Books.

Foulkes, S. H. (1964) *Therapeutic Group Analysis*. London: Allen and Unwin.

Foulkes, S. H. (1974 [1990]) My Philosophy in Psychotherapy. In Foulkes, E. (ed.) *Selected Papers, Psychoanalysis and Group Analysis*. London: Karnac.

Foulkes, S. H. (1975a [1990]) Problems of the Large Group. In Foulkes, E. (ed.) *Selected Papers, Psychoanalysis and Group Analysis*. London: Karnac.

Foulkes, S. H. (1975b) *Group-Analytic Psychotherapy: Method and Principles*. London: Gordon and Breach, Science Publishers Ltd.

Foulkes, S. H. and Anthony, E. J. (1957) *Group Psychotherapy: The Psychoanalytic Approach*, 2nd ed. London: Karnac.

Freire, P. (1996) *Pedagogy of the Oppressed*. Trans. M. B. Ramos. Toronto, CA: Penguin Books.

Freud, S. (1917 [1915]) *Mourning and Melancholia, Vol. 14 of the Standard Edition of the Complete Psychological Works of Sigmund Freud*. London: Vintage.

Freud, S. (1927) *The Future of an Illusion, Vol. 21 of The Standard Edition of the Complete Psychological Works of Sigmund Freud*. London: Vintage.

Gans, J. (2018) *Difficult Topics in Group Psychotherapy: My Journey from Shame to Courage*. London: Routledge.

Ghalaini, S. (2020) Another F***ing Growth Opportunity: Overcoming Islamophobia and the Enduring Impacts. *Studies in Gender and Sexuality*, 21(2): 99–103.

Glassgold, J. (2022) Research on Sexual Orientation Change Effort. In Haldeman, D. C. (ed.) *The Case Against Conversion "Therapy": Evidence, Ethics, and Alternatives*. Washington, DC: American Psychological Association.

Goffman, E. (1990 [1963]) *Stigma: Notes on the Management of Spoiled Identity*. London: Penguin Books.

Goldstein, K. (1939) *The Organism. A Holistic Approach to Biology Derived from Pathological Data in Man*. New York: American Book Company.

Grambal, A., et al. (2016) Self-Stigma in Borderline Personality Disorder – Cross-Sectional Comparison with Schizophrenia Spectrum Disorder, Major Depressive Disorder, and Anxiety Disorders. *Neuropsychiatric Disease and Treatment*, 12: 2439–2448, Dove Press.

Hamid, R. (2021) *Defining Islamophobia; A Contemporary Understanding of How Expressions of Muslimness Are Targeted, Muslim Council of Britain*, March. mcb.org.uk/islamophobia

Hartman, S. V. and Wilderson, F. B. (2003) The Position of the Unthought. *Qui Parle*, 13(2): 183–201.

Helbich, M. and Jabr, S. (2022) A Call for Social Justice and for a Human Rights Approach with Regard to Mental Health in the Occupied Palestinian Territories. *Health and Human Rights Journal*, 24(2): 305–318.

Hopper, E. and Weinberg, H. (eds.) (2011) *The Social Unconscious in Persons, Groups and Societies. Volume 1: Mainly Theory*. London: Karnac Books.

Ingoglia, P., et al. (2020) Secure Attachment and Individual Protective Factors Against Internalized Homophobia. *Journal of Gay & Lesbian Mental Health*, 24(2): 136–154. https://doi.org/10.1080/19359705.2019.1688746

Johnson, A. G. (2013) The Social Construction of Difference. In Adams, M., Blumenfeld, W. J., Castaneda, C. R., Hackman, H. W., Peters, M. L. and Zuniga, X. (eds.) *Readings for Diversity and Social Justice*, 3rd ed. London: Routledge, Taylor & Francis.

Kafai, S. (2013) The Mad Border Body; A Typical In-Betweeness. *Disability Studies Quarterly*, 33(1).

Kent, J. (2021) Scapegoating and the 'Angry Black Woman'. *Group Analysis*, 54(3): 354–371.

Klein, M. (1952 [1997]) Some Theoretical Conclusions Regarding the Emotional Life of the Infant. In *Envy and Gratitude and Other Works 1946–1963*. London: Vintage.

Koster, A. (2017) Mentalization, Embodiment, and Narrative: Critical Comments on the Social Ontology of Mentalization Theory. *Theory & Psychology*, 27(4): 458–476.

Kwarteng, J., et al. (2022) Misogynoir/Challenges in Detecting Intersectional Hate. *Social Network Analysis and Mining*, 12(1), Knowledge Media Institute, The Open University, UK. https://doi.org/10.1007/s13278-022-00993-7

Levy, K. N., et al. (2006) The Mechanisms of Change in the Treatment of Borderline Personality Disorder with Transference Focussed Psychotherapy. *Journal of Clinical Psychology*, 62(4): 481–501.

Lorde, A. (2019 [1984]) *Sister Outsider*. London: Penguin Modern Classics.

Luyton, P., Campbell, C. and Fonagy, P. (2019) Borderline Personality Disorder, Complex Trauma, and Problems with Self and Identity: A Social-Communicative Approach. *Journal of Personality*, 88: 88–105, Wiley Periodicals, Inc.

Manstead, A. (2018) The Psychology of Social Class: How Socioeconomic Status Impacts Thought, Feelings, and Behaviour. *British Journal of Social Psychology*, 57: 267–291, John Wiley & Sons.

Messina, K. E. (2019) *Misogyny, Projective Identification, and Mentalization: Psychoanalytic, Social, and Institutional Manifestations*. London: Routledge.

Milsom, C. (2021) *Defining Islamophobia; A Contemporary Understanding of How Expressions of Muslimness Are Targeted*, Muslim Council of Britain, March. mcb.org.uk/islamophobia

Mugglestone, L. (2003) *Talking Proper: The Rise of Accent as Social Symbol*, 2nd ed. Oxford: Oxford University Press.

Murchie, J. and Pang, J. (2018) Rental Housing Discrimination Across Protected Classes: Evidence from a Randomized Experiment. *Regional Science and Urban Economics*, 73: 170–179. https://doi.org/10.1016/j.regsciurbeco.2018.10.003 [Accessed online 28th February 2023].

Nayak, S. (2019) Occupation of Racial Grief, Loss as a Resource: Learning from 'The Combahee River Feminist Statement'. *Psychological Studies*, 64: 352–364.

Nayak, S. (2021) Racialized Misogyny: Response to 44th Foulkes Lecture. *Group Analysis*, 54(4): 520–527.

Nayak, S. (2022) An Intersectional Model of Reflection: Is Social Work Fit for Purpose in an Intersectionally Racist World? *Critical and Radical Social Work*, 10(2): 319–334.

Okri, B. (2016 [1991]) *The Famished Road*, 25th anniversary ed. London: Penguin Random House.

Parker, V. (2020) *A Group-Analytic Exploration of the Sibling Matrix. How Siblings Shape Our Lives*. London: Routledge, Taylor & Francis Group.

Piccini, J. (2021) *"A Fundamental Human Right?" Mixed-Race Marriage and the Meaning of Rights in the Postwar British Commonwealth, The Society for the Comparative Study of Society and History*. Cambridge: Cambridge University Press.

Pines, M. (1985) Psychic Development and the Group Analytic Situation. *Group*, 9(1): 24–37.

Roberts, A. L., et al. (2013) Does Maltreatment in Childhood Affect Sexual Orientation in Adulthood? *Archives of Sexual Behaviour*, 42(2): 161–171. https://doi.org/10.1007/s10508-012-0021-9

Ruggiero, I. (2012) *The Unreachable Object? Difficulties and Paradoxes in the Analytical Relationship with Borderline Patients*. London: Blackwell Publishing.

Sheehi, L. and Sheehi, S. (2022) *Psychoanalysis Under Occupation: Practicing Resilience in Palestine*. Oxford: Routledge.

Sheehy, C. and Nayak, S. (2020) Black Feminist Methods of Activisim Are the Tool for Global Social Justice and Peace. *Critical Social Policy*, 40(2): 234–257, Sage.

Shoshani, M., Shoshani, B. and Shinar, O. (2010) Fear and Shame in an Israeli Psychoanalyst and His Patient: Lessons Learned in Times of War. *Psychoanalytic Dialogues*, 20: 285–307.

Shuck, G. (2004) Conversational Performance and the Poetic Construction of an Ideology. *Language in Society*, 33: 195–222, Cambridge University Press.

Sousa, C., et al. (2013) Individual and Collective Dimensions of Resilience within Political Violence. *Trauma, Violence, & Abuse*, 14(3): 235–254.

Srour, R. (2015) Transference and Countertransference Issues During Times of Violent Political Conflict: The Arab Therapist – Jewish Patient Dyad. *Clinical Social Work Journal*, 43: 407–418.

Stacey, R. (2005) Social Selves and the Notion of the 'Group-as-a-Whole'. *Group*, 29(1), Eastern Group Psychotherapy Society, JSTOR Online [Accessed online 26th January 2020].

Stanghellini, G. and Rosfort, R. (2013) Borderline Depression a Desperate Vitality. *Journal of Consciousness Studies*, 20(7–8): 153–177.

Stobo, B. (2011) Race and the Social Unconscious, New Readings in Group Analysis Presentation. Adapted from dissertation for MSc in Group Analysis (2005) Location of Disturbance with a Focus on Race, Difference and Culture. *Presented at the Conference New Readings in Group Analysis,* London, United Kingdom.

Stoute, B. (2021) Black Rage: The Psychic Adaptation to the Trauma of Oppression. *Journal of the American Psychoanalytic Association*, 69(2): 259–290.

Subtirelu, N. (2015) 'She Does Have an Accent But . . .': Race and Language Ideology in Students' Evaluations of Mathematics Instructors on RateMyProfessors.com. *Language in Society*, 44: 35–62, Cambridge University Press.

Walker, N. (2021) *Neuroqueer Heresies: Notes on the Neurodiversity Paradigm*. Autistic Empowerment, and Postnormal Possibilities, Autonomous Press. ProQuest Ebook Central. http://ebookcentral.proquest.com/lib/ucl/detail.action?docID=6870963. Created from ucl on 2023–03–11 11:14:47.

Weegman, M. (2014) An Exclusionary Matrix: Degenerates, Addicts, Homosexuals. In *The World within the Group*. London: Karnac Books, pp. 103–118.

Woloshyn, V. and Savage, M. J. (2020) Features of YouTube Videos Produced by Individuals Who Self-Identify with Borderline Personality Disorder. *Digital Health*, 6: 1–11.

Zahrawi, S. (2020) The Arab-American Experience: Identity Negotiation in How Does It Feel to Be a Problem? *South Central Review*, 37(1): 121–137.

Zinkin, L. (1992) Borderline Distortions of Mirroring in the Group. *Group Analysis*, 25(1): 27–31.

Chapter 5

An Intersectional Response to the Intersectionality of Trauma

Suryia Nayak and Farideh Dizadji

Introduction

We begin this chapter with words from Audre Lorde. The implications of her words resonate with the mutually constitutive method and content of this chapter:

> *But for every real word spoken, for every attempt I had ever made to speak those truths for which I am still seeking, I had made contact with other women while we examined the words to fit a world in which we all believed, bridging our differences.*

(Lorde, 1977:41)

The structure and content of this chapter come from a continuing conversation between two women bridging our differences by speaking our intersectional truths. By examining the words to fit a world we believe in, we found commonality through the lens of intersectionality within the context of our group analytical thinking. We made contact with each other as women through 'theory as liberatory practice' (hooks, 1994:59). This was a co-productive experience where word by word, sentence by sentence ideas, feelings, and memories intersectionally created something we could not have predicted or known. Free floating conversation is central to group therapeutic approaches and, in particular, to Group Analysis (Brown, 1986). Moreover, conversation, as a method for change, is foundational to all movements for global social justice, solidarity, and mobilization against traumatic oppression (Sheehy and Nayak, 2018, 2020).

Our conversation reflects on three interrelated questions:

- Under the lens of intersectionality, what does it feel like to be traumatized, and is it possible to understand these feelings as intersectional?
- How do we relate to the intersectionality of trauma for a person or group?
- How can intersectionality enable an articulation of the basic aim of therapy with reference to trauma?

We argue that concepts of trauma need to be continually reinvented and re-understood within the political, social, and cultural contexts in which traumatization

DOI: 10.4324/9781003232216-6

occurs. More specifically, we argue that trauma is intersectional in its constitution and experience, and as such, the evolution of conceptual frameworks about trauma needs to be intersectional. The trauma experienced by refugees cannot be viewed simply in terms of subjective personal trauma but must be understood and worked with in terms of the political contexts that (re)produce trauma. Therefore, it is fitting that the anti-racist, feminist political theoretical methodology of intersectionality is used. Intersectionality has historical roots within the context and impact of racist, patriarchal trauma (Combahee River Collective, 1977). Hill-Collins and Bilge define intersectionality as

a way of understanding and analysing the complexity in the world, in people, and in human experience. The events and conditions of social and political life and the self can seldom be understood as shaped by one factor. They are shaped by many factors in diverse and mutually influencing ways.

(2016:2)

Farideh: The topic of 'Refugee and Trauma' is close to my heart and intertwined with my own personal experiences. I now wonder why it took me over 40 years to talk about it in the context of group analysis. On reflection, it seems working through those traumatic experiences, especially the ones caused by state organized violence, is a lifetime journey. Traumatized persons learn about their psychological and inner resilience capacity and how to detach themselves, unconsciously and consciously, from insufferable experiences in order just to survive. Defense mechanisms such as splitting, denial, and the false self become the norm to hide and protect the true self (Winnicott, 1990).

Over the last five years, I have been asked to contribute to the topic of Refugees and Trauma in different contexts. However, on all occasions, I have been ambivalent about accepting the invitation, feeling I have nothing to offer while working through some aspects of my fragmented Self in parallel. While the truth of the matter was otherwise.

I wonder why and why now? Contribution to this conversation is an attempt to understand something of these repeated parallel experiences. On reflection, it seems there are correlations between working through my trauma caused by state organized violence and my personal journey within the context of power, position, and privilege, which have been evolving over the years, in particular, in the last six years.

I am now wondering by submission of this published conversation, whether I can allow myself to 'to be exposed', to 'join in', 'to become part of', and 'to accept my own differences and the intersectionality of my multiple identities'? And finally, 'where do I choose to position myself or belong to'?

During the recent movement of Black Lives Matter, I became reconnected with the global social and political movements which I was part of during the 1960s and 1970s. I became interested and curious again about the development of Black Feminist theory and its movement and was introduced to the anti-racist, feminist political theoretical methodology of intersectionality and its connections and understanding in Group Analysis (Nayak, 2021).

While acknowledging the idea that the personal is social, it seems to me this reconnection, both literally and metaphorically, has been an indicative and continuous and parallel process of healing and working through traumatic personal, social, and political experiences. It is within this understanding that I asked you, Suryia to accompany me on the journey of this exploration.

I have been a political refugee in exile since 1984. The process of my recovery as a survivor of extreme organized violence has been slow, and it has taken me almost 41 years before I can now be able to feel the integration of what is so-called 'double-reality', or metaphorically, moving from a 'paranoid-schizoid position' to a 'depressive position' (Klein, 1946). On reflection, I have been living in two different worlds with two different identities: one, prior to the Iranian Revolution of 1979, when I was a citizen of the countries that I had chosen to live in, while on the other hand, a 'political refugee' who was not welcomed easily with her blue UNHCR political Refugee passport in any Western country. I became a citizen of the international diaspora, the refugee community, which was unknown to me prior to my forced flee.

I was born into a loving and caring family in Iran. From the age of 16, in the mid-1960s, until the time of the Iranian Revolution in 1979, I had been living and studying between two continents. I finished my education in Tehran and Los Angeles, and after completing a postgraduate degree at UCLA in 1976, I returned to Iran, where I became a lawyer in 1979.

I had been part of the international student movements of the 1960s and 1970s, and as a political/feminist activist, I got caught up in the fallout of the Iranian Revolution in the early eighties. Following the disappearance of my husband when our baby was only 45 days old and receiving the news of his execution 18 months later, I had to go underground. After two years in hiding, in the autumn of 1984, I was forced to flee Iran with my two-and-a-half-year-old son, through the mountains of Kurdistan in the Northwest of Iran to enter Turkey. A few months later, in December 1984, we were smuggled through East Berlin to West Berlin via Friedrichstrasse without any personal possessions. It was an extremely cold winter, but we were advised to enter without any belongings so as not to attract the attention of the German Police. I was granted political refugee status in West Berlin subsequently. In 1988, we resettled in London and went on to become British citizens.

Suryia: Firstly, I acknowledge your courage in speaking out about your experience. The word 'courage' has in it 'cor' – the Latin word for heart – so that 'courage' comes to mean 'inner strength from the heart'. Secondly, I am reminded of the words of Audre Lorde, 'silence will not protect' (Lorde, 1977:41), but how when to speak and how to speak is a process of navigation analogous to journeying through treacherous mountains holding the child within. Here, I am reminded of Volkan's (2003) idea of perennial mourners to describe the specific situation of refugees and the ongoing psychological journey of intersecting losses. The question, 'I wonder why it took me over 40 years to talk about it in the context of group analysis?' says something about the nature of silence, of time, and calls for a re-examination of ambivalence in the context of trauma generally and more specifically for political refugees. How do we understand the expression of ambivalence in trauma? An intersectional lens on ambivalence in trauma exposes ambivalence as a negotiation of internal territories of rejection and acceptance, which, for a political refugee, is the struggle of internal citizenship. Ambivalence is not something to get rid of or resolve, rather, it could be likened to a territory to reside in where the struggle is actually the site of productive healing (Forrest and Nayak, 2021).

I am not a refugee. The roots and experiences of my trauma are different, but I know that intersectionality, particularly emotional intersectional, continues to be instrumental in my understanding of trauma (Nayak, 2015:85–116, 2021). In a world constituted and contingent upon divisions, binaries, and fragmentation, an emotional depressive position (Klein, 1946) of intersectionality is difficult to inhabit.

My parents were first-generation immigrants who never felt at home in England. My mother is from a large Irish Catholic family and grew up in Co. Wicklow, Ireland. My father, now deceased, was from a large Hindu family and grew up in Odisha, India. Back in 1990, when my mother visited my father's family in India, she was the first white person to have ever been inside the village, and to this day, she is still the only white outsider to step foot in the village. My parents shared a migratory experience of moving from homelands subjected to colonialism. They shared the common experience of 'No Irish, No Blacks, No dogs'. I was born into an intergenerational social unconscious of colonialism and racism. I have carried this my whole life (Biran, 2014; Hopper, 2003a; Weinberg, 2007). As Blackwell points out, '[t]he colonial patterns of relationship remain deep in our social unconscious' (2003:456). Trauma knows no temporal borders; trauma has no adherence to time. Intergenerational, historical trauma is transmitted unconsciously to amplify our individual, community, and collective lived experiences of trauma. In terms of working with trauma in group therapy, I am reminded of Kleij's evocative reflection that '[a]ll kinds of ghosts hover around the physical boundaries of the group' (1983:77). Inhabiting the ghosts of trauma whilst in the process of inhabiting the present is a pivotal task for people are traumatized; a process of multiple habitation that is especially painful for refugees who have extreme trauma. My group analytic journey has enabled me to see the malignant mirroring of 'No Irish, No Blacks, No dogs' in group therapy, supervision, and large group experiences. My/our identities are products of contexts operating across political, social, and cultural temporal and spatial dimensions. Indeed, 'in order to understand the transference, it must be contextualised, that is, related to other categories of events which stand in specified relationships to the transference in terms of time and social psychological space' (Hopper, 1982:139). The multiple interconnected dimensions of context can be understood as contextual-situated intersectionality (Montenegro et al., 2018).

My/our developing and frequently inconsistent capacity to hold intersectionality on an emotional internal level is pivotal to the extent to which, in the words of Audre Lorde, we can

> *lie down with the different parts of ourselves, so that we can in fact learn to respect and honor the different parts of each other so that we in fact can learn how to use them, moving toward something that needs to be done, that has never been done before.*

(Abod, 1987:158)

Enabling the intersectionality of our multiple identities is imperative to psychological well-being. Psychological intersectionality of our multiple differences shapes where we are positioned and our sense of belonging.

Intersectionality was born out of trauma to tackle trauma. Specifically, intersectionality was born out of the struggles of Black women's traumatic lived experience of the interconnection and interdependency of racism and misogyny in the context of colonial capitalism (Hill Collins and Bilge, 2016; Nayak and Robbins, 2018; Phoenix and Pattynama, 2006; Yuval-Davis, 2006). The traumatic psychological disturbance of simultaneous multiple oppression 'can never be wholly confined to a person in isolation' (Foulkes, 1948:127). Sojourner Truth's intersectional plea for humanity, 'Ain't I a woman' (1851), endures the present geopolitical world and pervades our group therapy spaces. Intersectionality holds an enduring international perspective refusing belonging to one space or single axis perspective ideologically, contextually, and emotionally. In terms of group therapy,

> *[w]e tend to forget the powerful influence of contextual society on our small groups. We tend to share the illusion that our analytic room exists in a kind of empty space, whereas in fact the foundation matrix always envelopes the dynamic matrix of the group and it penetrates the small group's setting, as seen in many processes of equivalence.*

(Biran, 2018:261)

Farideh: Focussing on the question of how do we relate to the intersectionality of trauma for a person or group? According to Harré and Gillet (1994), to have a sense of identity is to be quadruply located: in space, in time, in agency, and in the social world. This intersectionality of locations positions all our personal histories in a particular web of social relationships and provides a sense of existing at a given moment as part of an unfolding collective history. The 'wound' of psychosocial trauma has social roots, and its nature is sustained and recreated in social interactions. A basic aim of group therapy is to (re)create conditions for social interactions. Trauma impacts the basis of collective existence and identity. Intersectionality enables articulation of the socio-historical realities where trauma is inflicted and where it gains meaning while placing symptoms in the particular features of each individual. Intersectionality acknowledges the dynamic simultaneous intersection of socio-historical realities and symptoms.

Intersectionality concerns identity and contexts across temporal and spatial dimensions, which are particular aspects of the intersectional experience of being a refugee and exiled. The emphasis in intersectionality on deconstructing vectors of identity to understand the interconnection and interdependency of these vectors is vital to the process of reconstruction of identity and the way in which notions of the past are invoked to achieve continuity.

The task of group or individual therapy is to understand that in order to preserve the temporal dimension of the self, the radical rupture of exile must be signified in light of the present reality of the subjects. This construction of continuity, which takes place in communicative practices and positions the subject regarding their reality while endowing them with a series of properties that condition their existential possibilities. The self, thus, appears not as a thing but as a dynamic subject-position constructed in the communicative practices within social interaction. Multiple intersecting subject-positions emerge in the co-creation of narratives through group therapy. Different social frameworks inside and outside of group therapy constitute the position through which the subject makes sense of their experiences. For example, the transition from exiled to refugee appears as a reorganization of the axes that shape the subject's identity, thereby engendering or cancelling different existential possibilities. In the case of the refugees interviewed, narratives about life in the home country position them as agents endowed with initiative, while the status of refugees in the country of asylum places them mainly as victims of persecution, threats, and objects of other's initiative and power.

Suryia: Over and over again, the issue of location appears central to intersectionality and, more specifically, to an intersectional articulation of the trauma of being a political refugee. Intersectionality is an anti-border theory and methodology that refuses ideas of location demarcated by borders. Geopolitical borders, including ideological borders based on hegemony that (re)produce conflict and war, are central to the refugee trauma. Trauma-informed therapeutic approaches must be vigilant to conscious and unconscious gravitation towards the recreations of psychic borders. For the therapist, this means holding professional ethical borders of therapeutic practice that sustain safe containment whilst holding an eye to the (re) enactments of trauma-producing borders within transference relational interactions. Blackwell reminds us that '[c]rossing boundaries involves not only boundaries of geography, nationality, culture, class, 'race' and gender, but addressing the boundaries in our individual and collective minds, and it is usually those boundaries that are the hardest to cross' (2018:313).

An intersectional group therapy approach to the location of disturbance opens curiosity of location as a multiple undecidable situation. The location of disturbance is in the intersection of multiple collisions travelling across multiple axes. Radhakrishnan explains, '[t]he politics of location is productive . . . it makes one location vulnerable to the claims of another and enables multiple contested readings of the one reality from a variety of locations and positions' (2000:56–57).

Radhakrishnan's analysis is congruent with Foulkes' insistence of location as a dynamic 'process' (Foulkes, 1986:131). This dynamic process troubles demarcations of the beginning and end of what is inside and outside a border. The implications can be highly anxiety-provoking in terms of being 'vulnerable' to the 'Other', whether that is an internalized 'Other' within self or the 'Other' within external social relations. Locational intersectionality is vital to understanding the intersectional experience of trauma, what it feels like to be traumatized, and how to understand these feelings as intersectional.

I have argued that 'our understanding of intersectionality is enriched by psychanalytic thinking and our understanding of psychoanalytic group thinking is enriched by intersectionality – a kind of reciprocity or reciprocal praxis' (Nayak, 2021:343). Group therapy is formed by reciprocal exchanges between the intersectional selves of the people in the group. The therapeutic impetus of groups lies within reciprocity and intersectionality. Whilst reciprocity and intersectionality are distinct concepts in their own right, they share foundational mutually constitutive characteristics, such as open fluidity of borders and relations of exchange. There is no reciprocity without intersectionality, and there is no intersectionality without reciprocity. Enabling internal reciprocity for the traumatized individual through social exchanges of reciprocity within group therapy is an intersectional articulation of the basic aim of therapy. However, if 'all exchange enhances relations of exchange' (O'Neill, 1999:133), we need an eye to power in relations of exchange. Here, the lens of intersectionality, with its direct focus on power, enables scrutiny of the dynamics of give and take. Definitions of reciprocity stress the element of mutual benefit. However, constructions of mutual benefit or the perimeters of reciprocity depend on positions of privilege and power. But, and this is precisely why intersectionality was coined by Crenshaw (1989), well-intentioned anti-discriminatory, feminist, and anti-racist frameworks to enhance relations of power exchange are flawed when they are 'grounded in experiences that actually represent only a subset of a much more complex phenomenon' (Crenshaw, 1989:140). Being on the receipt end of 'relations of exchange' that disavow the complexity of experience, position, and context, where experience is 'theoretically erased/imports its own theoretical limitations' (ibid.), is traumatic. Herein lies the necessity for an intersectional, trauma-informed group therapy approach.

Intersectional Trauma Work

Farideh: The Greek etymology of the word 'trauma' literally means 'wound' (Garland, 1998:9). Going beyond the medical application of 'wound' as the piercing of the bodily envelope, a psychological trauma metaphorically denotes a wound to the psychological envelope that functions to filter excess stimulation. In trauma, the unthinkable or that which has necessarily been filtered out becomes a concrete, unbearable reality. Garland explains

> *a traumatic event is one which . . . breaks through or overrides the discriminatory, filtering process . . . the mind is flooded. . . . Something very violent feels*

as though it happened internally, and this mirrors the violence that is felt to have happened, or indeed actually happened, in the external world.

(Garland, 1998:10–11)

The result is a 'loss in symbolic thinking' (Garland, 1998:17). A loss in belief, trust, and capacity in the symbolic 'what if' quality of thinking because the unimaginable 'what if' has happened. For the political refugee, the concrete and psychic experience of violation results in an amplified loss of the symbolic 'what if' causing existential disorientation (Tucker, 2011).

In understanding trauma theory, we need to understand and distinguish between the traumatic situation, the trauma, and the symptoms resulting from trauma whilst recognizing and identifying their interdependence and interconnections. A traumatic situation could be defined as an event or series of events of extreme violence that occur within a social context, such as war. However, although such a traumatic situation is required, it is not enough of a condition for trauma to occur. Similarly, trauma suggests the destruction of an individual and/or group but not necessarily its symptoms. The classified symptoms (known as PTSD) can remain with the survivor of a traumatic situation.

With reference to the intrapsychic dynamics of trauma, fragmentation, as a conscious and unconscious defence mechanism, is a central characteristic and can only be overcome within a close relationship that recognizes and accepts the destruction that has occurred and helps construct a space in which symbolization can take place. The intersectional experiences of refugees 'cannot be treated as "independent variables" because the oppression of each is inscribed within the other – is constituted by, and is constitutive of the other' (Brah, 1996:109).

Ferenczi states that '[w]hat is traumatic is the unforeseen, the unfathomable, the incalculable. . . . Unexpected, external threat, the sense of which one cannot grasp, is unbearable' (Ferenczi, 1932:171). Ferenczi's extensive oeuvre on trauma points to psychic 'fragmentation' as a defense in surviving traumatic situations. Trauma, at its core, feels like extreme suffering and torments of fear that lead to the psychological experience of death, which means that a basic split has to happen (Soreanu, 2018). Part of a person stays dead, while another part begins to function again (Lifton, 1973). This is what I had to do in order to not have a breakdown and carry on with my political and personal responsibilities as a mother and political feminist activist.

The task is to overcome the fragmentation to overcome trauma. However, it is nearly impossible to deal with trauma in such a linear manner because 'within' the traumatic experience, there are only pains, no words, and a constrained capacity for thinking reflectively. 'Outside' of trauma, thinking works, and words exist, but without being totally connected to the traumatic experiences. Here, I speak from my personal experience of trauma; we need to understand this double-reality: on one side, there is a person who can talk about, think about, and even tell us about what happened to them. On the other side, we have a person lost in the experience of death and terror, for whom there are no words to explain their experience. The task of therapy is to work through this 'double-reality' and bring them together, to contain the fear, and to offer an authentic but sufficiently secure space to begin the process of reintegration.

Suryia: I am reminded that where we speak or do not speak, where we reveal self or hide 'are inseparable as a constant opposition, reference, interruption, and container, to the other' (Barnes, 2015:27). Picking up on the themes of fragmentation, double reality, language, and silence, I offer the following vignette:

> *'K', a political refugee who was a boy soldier in the 1990s civil war in Afghanistan and a patient in group therapy, found it impossible to tell the group why he was late and absent from group sessions. In his personal relationship, 'K' also found it impossible to tell his partner why he was late, where he was going, and the content of his day-to-day activities when he was apart from her. 'K' would leave the family home without a 'goodbye' or notice of going out and without any detail of the purpose of going out. The therapy group and his partner experienced this inability to give words to his actions as a lack of commitment, lack of accountability, and lack of responsibility. However, nothing could have been further from the truth. As a boy soldier in Afghanistan, 'K' was trained, as a literal matter of life and death, to keep silent about his whereabouts. 'K' had witnessed the inhumane, brutal consequences of torture and execution that his peers, boy soldiers who did not adhere to the rule of silence, suffered. 'K' was now faced with the excruciatingly painful double reality of identity and context as a soldier in a civil war and a civilian refugee in the UK.*

In this vignette, the traumatized political refugee 'K' and those close to him in therapy and personal relationships struggled to hold a psychic intermediate (Walshe, 2006) outsider-insider position. For 'K', the experience of double reality necessitated split fragmentation or attacks on linking (Bion, 1959). Biran explains that 'violent attacks injure our mental hygiene. Self-defence against such an unbearable pain often entails inter-psychic disengagement, intra-psychic encapsulation (Hopper, 2003b) and social psychic retreats (Mojovic, 2011)' (Biran, 2018:263). This is precisely where and why emotional intersectionality is vital. Emotional intersectionality attends to the function and production of psychic divisions founded on the imperative that '[w]hat is inside is outside, the social is not external but very much internal too and penetrates the innermost being of the individual's personality' (Foulkes, 1973:227). An intersectional lens on intrapsychic defenses of fragmentation that are central to the intrapsychic dynamics of trauma prompts us to refuse 'mutually exclusive categories of identity, experience, and analysis' (Nayak, 2021:343). The challenge in holding an intersectional mindset for group therapists is

> *that it is much easier to visualize a unitary particle, and nigh impossible to visualize a field. A particle, an individual, is bounded and looks infinite to the eye. This makes it easier for us to formulate thoughts about it, relate it to other*

things. . . . In contrast a field is so much more amorphous, it is fluctuating continuum with no end in sight.

(Dalal, 1998:221)

Notwithstanding the challenges, and to be clear, intersectionality is immensely difficult to sustain emotionally, intersectionality enables exploration of psychic boundary events (Minh-ha, 2011) where boundaries are not merely demarcations of division but actual spaces of experience. Within group-therapy, it is the sensitive exploration of the 'event' of space of fragmentation, in terms of ruptures and disturbances or rigid where the opportunity for reparation lies.

Farideh: I find the following frames useful: Bettelheim's idea of 'extreme traumatisation', Khan's idea of 'cumulative trauma', and Keilson's idea of 'sequential traumatization'.

Bettelheim (1943) wrote about his time in a concentration camp and suggested the need for a new term to describe the experiences he and his fellow prisoners had suffered:

[W]hat characterised it most was its inescapability, its uncertain duration, but potentiality for life; the fact that nothing about it was predictable; that one's very life was in jeopardy at every moment and that one could do nothing about it.

(Bettelheim, 1943:418; see also Levi, 1959).

Picking up on the 'unpredictable' quality and experience of trauma reminds me of the experience I had with a political prisoner, K, who had nightmares regularly for more than 35 years. K was a teenager when she was arrested for her political activities during the Iranian Revolution of 1979. For a while, we shared a bedroom, and every night, I was woken up by her screams while she slept. One night, after waking her up while she was experiencing a nightmare, she told me her violent dreams related to the time she was in prison and tortured when she was 19 years old. For months, she was kept in a small caste-type box for up to 20 hours a day. She said, 'It was like a baby grave'. The trauma of imprisonment and torture are unpredictable in that the forms of inhumanity experienced are unable to be predicted in thought and feeling, rendering them unthinkable and unbounded. The inescapability of the trauma of imprisonment and torture, visiting during waking and sleeping, with no predicated duration, needs to be responded to with a therapeutic approach that does not set limits on duration. An intersectional response to trauma actively works with the unbounded unpredictability of trauma because intersectionality enables an opening up of the metaphorical caste-type box of constricted constructions to reveal the interconnected and interdependent uncertainty of lines of experience and context. No trauma is a bounded site of experience. All trauma is part of an interconnected web of experience.

Bettelheim was the first to clearly illustrate that traumatization resulting from a man-made disaster could not be categorized in the usual psychiatric or psychoanalytical language, and the term 'extreme situation' to describe his experiences, and eventually, the term 'extreme traumatizations' was developed. The word 'extreme' conveyed the special nature of the trauma, which can be applied to the experience of asylum seekers and refugees today, that it could not be compared to other types of traumatic events such as accidents, an earthquake, or a heart attack, and cannot be understood by a diagnostic model of medicine. Extreme trauma is produced in contexts of political oppression, and psychotherapeutic responses need to have explicit relevance to contexts of political oppression. Here is precisely why intersectionality as a theory of liberatory practice is necessary because intersectionality was born out of the socio-political oppression of Black women, including slavery, lynching, and incarceration. Intersectionality names and frames the extreme situation of being in danger of life because of identity and position.

'Extreme traumatization' is an individual and collective process that refers to and is dependent on a given social context, a process of interdependency between the social and the psychological dimensions of existence. Extreme traumatization exceeds the capacity of the individual and of social structures to respond adequately to the intersectionality of the social and psychological impact. The aim of extreme traumatization is the destruction of the individual and of their sense of belonging to society and social activities. Extreme traumatization is characterized by a structure of power within the society that is based on the elimination of some of its members by other members of the same society. The process of extreme traumatization is not limited in time and develops sequentially (Becker and Castillo, 1990).

Masud Khan (1977) followed Freud's idea about trauma that occur as a result of several experiences and developed the concept of 'cumulative trauma'. According to Khan, as explained by Becker:

> [T]rauma can be a product of a series of individually non-traumatic experiences, which develop and accumulate within an interactive framework and finally lead to a breakdown. These ideas are highly important because, although initially limited to the mother-child relationship, they transfer the emphasis from the trauma to the traumatic situation. This converts the event into a process and, without denying the intrapsychic, would focus on the importance of the interactive framework.

(Becker, 2004)

An intersectional approach to cumulative trauma would explicitly concentrate on the nature of the interactions of multiple experiences. Importantly, intersectionality focuses attention on the play of power within the interaction of traumatic experiences.

Bettelheim's and Khan's ideas were later developed in the 1970s by Hans Keilson's concept of 'sequential traumatization' (Keilson, 1992 [1979]). This concept was developed from his follow-up study of Jewish war orphans in the Netherlands. However, it has application to contemporary global refugees' traumatic situations, for example, Palestinian, Afghan, Syrian, and Ukrainian refugees, their families, and children.

Keilson suggests a radical change in the understanding of trauma. Instead of an event that has consequences, the focus is on the process. The focus is on the process of the changing traumatic situation; this process produces a kind of internal framework that organizes our understanding of trauma. This is extremely important in explaining why trauma continues, even when the active persecution has stopped. We are, therefore, able to understand not only why clients might develop symptoms immediately after the original event but also why they might do so 20, 30, or 40 years later. Keilson's framework illustrates that since there is no 'post' in trauma, but only a continuing traumatic process, the helpers (the people who deal with the survivors) are also always part of the traumatic situation and do not operate outside of it.

Keilson's framework of 'sequential traumatization' can be used in different cultural and political settings. It does not define a fixed set of symptoms or situations but actually only invites one to look closely at a specific historical process; it allows the quality and the quantity of the traumatic sequences to be very different in various contexts. In addition, Yoa'd Ghanadry-Hakim, Palestine Counseling Centre, Beit Hanina Branch (2020) argues that there is no 'post' in trauma by rejecting the term PTSD in understanding and working with refugees' trauma experiences, including Palestinian refugees, as their trauma has been ongoing experiences; within this frame, she continues, and suggests that PTSD should be replaced by CTSD – Continuous Trauma Stress Disorder.

In each different social context, people should be given room to create their own definitions of trauma, and the basic aim of psychotherapy with trauma is understanding the configurations of individual and collective unconscious frameworks for managing trauma. A sequential traumatization model of understanding trauma does not focus on symptoms but on the intersecting sequential developments of the traumatic situation. Although it will always be important to register the specific symptoms of a client, our primary approach must focus on the repressive experiences and their intersectionality.

An intersectional framing of any traumatic experience or circumstance recognizes that the traumatic condition and context is never one dimensional but has multiple parts, and different facets of a trauma will manifest itself psychologically and physically or materially in different interconnected and interdependent ways.

The recovery of extremely traumatized persons neither begins nor ends in a therapist's room. However, therapy may become the first safe social space in which survivors of extreme violence might begin to think about their pains. The relatively safe space of therapy permits us to explore some of the key issues of trauma, such as understanding the feeling of a traumatized person, finding ways to relate to that person, and what we are hoping to achieve.

Conclusion

Psychotherapists working with trauma that is a result of the extreme situation of political imprisonment, torture, and exile need to guard against 'a tendency to interpret people's experiences of existing oppressive social structures, as mani-festations of projection, rather than take them at face value and challenge them' (Dalal, 2015:362). The physical reality of inhumanity that political refugees have been actually subject to are concrete material manifestations of abuses of power, position, and privilege that cannot be understood through a single axis of the psy-chological or unconscious dynamic. The situation of the trauma of political refu-gees has to be understood as the convergence of compound, simultaneous, multiple realities that need a methodological theory adequate to handle this complexity. Whilst systemic or system theory-focused models of psychotherapy work with interacting multiplicity or dynamic processes of multiple factors, they usually fail to explicitly name and frame the political machinations of abuses of power, privi-lege, and power.

Under the lens of intersectionality, what does it feel like to be traumatized, and is it possible to understand these feelings as intersectional? Davis and Zarkov (2017:137) argue that 'intersectionality is taken up as a way to understand both the specific dynamics of social divisions and the ways they are intertwined and mutually constitutive, but also the possibilities they may engender for solidarity, resistance and transformation'. Trauma is a knot of intertwined psycho-socio-political dynamics that cannot be separated out into categorized, experienced, or linear formulations of imprisonment + torture + exile +++. The overwhelming feeling of trauma may be managed in terms of living a double reality or multiple versions of self, but the key word here is 'managed', for what is overwhelming is the intersection of multiple parts. The temporal dimension of intersectionality knows no past, present, or future but rather understands that the intersectional experience of past, present, and future is greater than the sum of any chronol-ogy. The spatial dimension of intersectionality enables therapeutic political exploration of the mutually constitutive dynamics of death and life, forgetting and remembering, finding and hiding (Becker, 1975). Here, Baker's words have resonance:

> *No one wants to recognise themselves in images of destruction, but traumatised persons have no choice. They can try to forget but this never works. The terror is part of them. The question is not does the person want to look at the terror, but how will a person look at this terror? Will he or she do so alone? In nightmares? Or will there be a space of sharing, of interaction with others, where death can become part of a living relationship?*
> (Becker, 2004:7–8; see also Hirschberger, 2018)

How do we relate to the intersectionality of trauma for a person or group? An intersectional framing of any traumatic experience or circumstance recognizes that the traumatic condition and context are never one dimensional but have multiple parts, and different facets of a trauma will manifest itself psychologi-cally and physically or materially in different interconnected and interdepend-ent ways. The recovery of extremely traumatized persons neither begins nor ends in a therapist's room. However, therapy may become the first safe social space in which survivors of extreme violence might begin to think about their pains. For the relatively safe space of therapy to give room for political activists to communicate something of their own, it is imperative that the psychotherapist has the psychological capacity to bear witness to the testimony of a survivor of trauma and be able to withstand being symbolically equated with the perpetrator of violence (Rohr, 2002). The psychotherapist working with traumatized political refugees needs robust supervision to inevitably embodied psychic countertransference reactions to unbearable, unpredictable mental images, dreams, and impulses. If extreme traumatization aims to annihilate an individual or group, it is inevitable that entering the psychic world of extreme traumatization and offering the self as a psychic vessel of emotional containment will bring the psychotherapist into close proximity to a sense of annihilation. Traumatized political refugees, people who have experienced cumulative extreme trauma, do not need or want pity or sympathy and will quickly sense being fitted into formulaic trauma models; after all, resistance to the imposition of ideological frameworks is a defining characteristic of political refugees and the grounds for punishing consequences. In essence, 'methodologically . . . we have to work harder to acquire and use multiple approaches' (McDowell, 2008:504).

How can intersectionality enable an articulation of the basic aim of therapy with reference to trauma? The basic aim of group therapy articulated through intersectionality could be explained through the simile that Foulkes uses to describe the relational process of group analytic therapy:

suppose you have to wash a number of dirty shirts together, and the water is not even clean and perhaps you have not even soap . . . even then you can get the shirts reasonably clean, albeit you add dirt to dirt, by using them for mutual friction upon each other.

(Foulkes, 1948:29)

Dirty shirts and dirt could be understood as the psychic disturbance of the intersectional effects of trauma. Here, the group analytic situation where the collective 'mutual friction' of individual member's disturbance is transformed would attend to the trauma 'constrained by social events' (Hopper, 1982:153). Here, intersectionality would concentrate on how 'the politics of location brings forward a whole host of identifications and associations around concepts of place, placement, displacement; location, dis-location; memberment, dis-memberment; citizenship, alienness; boundaries, barriers, transportations; peripheries, cores and centers' (Boyce Davies, 1994:153). An intersectional articulation of the function of psychotherapy, in the form of group or individual therapy, foregrounds the political axes of power. An intersectional articulation of psychotherapy refuses the idea that therapy is politically neutral.

References

Abod, J. (1987) Audre Lorde: A Radio Profile. In Wylie Hall, J. (ed.) (2004) *Conversations with Audre Lorde*. Jackson: University Press of Mississippi, pp. 158–163.

Barnes, C. (2015) Speaking with Silence. An Exploration of Silence and Its Relationship to Speech in Analytic Groups. *Group Analysis*, 48(1): 12–30. https://doi.org/10.1177/0533316414566160

Becker, D. (2004) Dealing with Consequences of Organised Violence in Trauma Work. In *Berghof Handbook for Conflict Transformation*. Berlin: Berghof Foundation.

Becker, D. and Castillo, M. I. (1990) *Procesos de Tramatizacion extrema y posibilidaes de reparacion*, Unpublished Paper, Instituto Latinoamericano de Salud Mental y Derechos Humanos, Santiago, Chile.

Becker, E. (1975) *Birth and Death of Meaning*. New York: Simon and Schuster.

Bettelheim, B. (1943) Individual and Mass Behaviour in Extreme Situations. *Journal of Abnormal and Social Psychology*, 38: 447–452.

Bion, W. R. (1959) Attacks on Linking. *International Journal of Psycho-Analysis*, 40(5–6): 308–315.

Biran, H. (2014) The Intersubjective and Social Unconscious are Inseparable. *Group Analysis*, 47(3): 283–292. https://doi.org/10.1177/0533316414545285

Biran, H. (2018) The 'Invisible Refugee'. *Group Analysis*, 51(3): 261–270. https://doi.org/10.1177/0533316418794656

Blackwell, D. (2003) Colonialism and Globalization: A Group-Analytic Perspective. *Group Analysis*, 36(4): 445–463. https://doi.org/10.1177/0533316403364002

Blackwell, D. (2018) Cultural Transition, Negation and the Social Unconscious1. *Group Analysis*, 51(3): 304–314. https://doi.org/10.1177/0533316418791102

Boyce Davies, C. (1994) *Black Women, Writing and Identity: Migrations of the Subject*. London: Routledge.

Brah, A. (1996) *Cartographies of Diaspora: Contesting Identities*. Abingdon: Routledge.

Brown, D. G. (1986) Dialogue for Change. *Group Analysis*, 19(1): 25–38. https://doi.org/10.1177/0533316486191004

The Combahee River Collective (1977) A Black Feminist Statement. In James, J. and Sharpley-Whiting, T. D. (eds.) (2000) *The Black Feminist Reader*. Oxford: Blackwell Publishers Ltd., pp. 261–270.

Crenshaw, K. (1989) Demarginalizing the Intersection of Race and Sex: A Black Feminist Critique of Antidiscrimination Doctrine, Feminist Theory and Antiracist Politics. *The University of Chicago Legal Forum. Feminism in the Law: Theory, Practice and Criticism*, 1989(Article 8): 139–167. https://chicagounbound.uchicago.edu/uclf/vol1989/iss1/8.

Dalal, F. (1998) *Taking the Group Seriously, Towards a Post-Foulkesian Analytic Theory*. London: Jessica Kingsley Publishers.

Dalal, F. (2015) Group Analytic Training and the Social Context: Who Is Influencing Whom? *Group Analysis*, 48(3): 349–367.

Davis, K. and Zarkov, D. (2017) EJWS Retrospective on Intersectionality. *European Journal of Women's Studies*, 24(4): 313–320. https://doi.org/10.1177/1350506817719393

Ferenczi, S. (1932 [1988]) *The Clinical Diary of Sandor Ferenczi*. Ed. J. Dupont, Trans. M. Balint and N. Z. Jackson. Cambridge, MA: Harvard University Press.

Forrest, A. and Nayak, S. (2021) 'Should I Stay or Should I Go?' Group-Analytic Training: Inhabiting the Threshold of Ambivalence Is a Matter of Power, Privilege and Position. *Group Analysis*, 54(1): 55–68. https://doi.org/10.1177/0533316420947999

Foulkes, S. H. (1948 [1984]) *Introduction to Group-Analytic Psychotherapy: Studies in the Social Interaction of Individuals and Groups*. London: Karnac. [Original publication, London: Heinemann].

Foulkes, S. H. (1973) The Group as Matrix of the Individual's Mental Life. In Foulkes, E. (ed.) (1990) *Selected Papers of SH Foulkes: Psychoanalysis and Group Analysis*. London: Karnac Books, pp. 223–233.

Foulkes, S. H. (1986) *Group Analytic Psychotherapy: Methods and Principles*. London: Karnac Books.

Garland, C. (1998) *Understanding Trauma: A Psychoanalytical Approach*. London: Gerald Duckworth Press & Co.

Harré, R. and Gillet, G. (1994) *The Discursive Mind*. London: Sage.

Hill Collins, P. and Bilge, S. (2016) *Intersectionality: Key Concepts*. Cambridge: Polity Press.

Hirschberger, G. (2018) Collective Trauma and the Social Construction of Meaning. *Frontiers in Psychology*, 9, 1441. https://doi.org/10.3389/fpsyg.2018.01441

hooks, b. (1994) *Teaching to Transgress: Education as the Practice of Freedom*. New York: Routledge.

Hopper, E. (1982) The Problem of Context. *Group Analysis*, 15(2): 136–157.

Hopper, E. (2003a) *The Social Unconscious: Selected Papers*. London: Jessica Kingsley Publishers.

Hopper, E. (2003b) *Traumatic Experience in the Unconscious Life of Groups*. London: Jessica Kingsley Publishers.

Keilson, H. (1992) *Sequential Traumatization in Children*. Jerusalem: Magnes Press, Hebrew University [First published in German in 1979].

Khan, M. (1977) Das Kumulative Trauma. In Khan, M. (ed.) *Selbsterfahrung in de Therapie*. Muchen: Kindle Verlag.

Kleij, G. V. D. (1983) The Setting of the Group. *Group Analysis*, 16(1): 75–80. https://doi.org/10.1177/053331648301600108

Klein, M. (1946) Notes on Some Schizoid Mechanisms. *The International Journal of Psychoanalysis*, 27: 99–110.

Levi, P. (1959) *Survival in Auschwitz*. New York: The Orion Press.

Lifton, R. J. (1973) The Sense of Immortality: On Death and the Continuity of Life. *The American Journal of Psychoanalysis*, 33: 3–15. https://doi.org/10.1007/BF01872131

Lorde, A. (1977) The Transformation of Silence into Language and Action. In Lorde, A. (ed.) (1984) *Sister Outsider: Essays and Speeches*. Trumansburg: The Crossing Press, pp. 40–44.

McDowell, L. (2008) Thinking Through Work: Complex Inequalities, Constructions of Difference and Trans-National Migrants. *Progress in Human Geography*, 32(4): 491–507.

Minh-ha, T. T. (2011) *Elsewhere, Within Here: Immigration, Refugeeism and the Boundary Event*. New York: Routledge.

Mojovic, M. (2011) Manifestations of Psychic Retreats in Social Systems. In Hopper, E. and Weinberg, H. (eds.) (2003) *The Social Unconscious in Persons, Groups, and Societies*, London: Routledge, pp. 209–234.

Montenegro, M., Pujol, J. and Nayak, S. (2018) Contextual Intersectionality: A Conversation. In Nayak, S. and Robbins, R. (eds.) *Intersectionality in Social Work: Activism and Practice in Context*. Abingdon: Routledge.

Nayak, S. (2015) *Race, Gender and the Activism of Black Feminist Theory: Working with Audre Lorde*. Abingdon: Routledge.

Nayak, S. (2021) Black Feminist Intersectionality Is Vital to Group Analysis: Can Group Analysis Allow Outsider Ideas In? *Group Analysis*. https://doi.org/10.1177/0533316421997767

Nayak, S. and Robbins, R. (eds.) (2018) *Intersectionality in Social Work: Activism and Practice in Context*. Abingdon: Routledge.

O'Neill, J. (1999) What Gives (with Derrida)? *European Journal of Social Theory*, 2(2): 131–145. https://doi.org/10.1177/13684319922224374

Phoenix, A. and Pattynama, P. (2006) 'Intersectionality.' Special Issue on 'Intersectionality'. *European Journal of Women's Studies*, 13: 187–192.

Radhakrishnan, R. (2000) Postmodernism and the Rest of the World. In Afzal-Khan, F. and Seshadri-Crooks, K. (eds.) *The Pre-occupation of Postcolonial Studies*. Durham: Duke University Press, pp. 37–70.

Rohr, E. (2002) Lost Shadows – Migrants, Refugees and Social Class: A Group-Analytic Challenge. *Group Analysis*, 35(3): 424–436. https://doi.org/10.1177/0533316402035003614

Sheehy, C. and Nayak, S. (2018) A Feminist Trade Unionist Response to the Academy as a Workplace: A Conversation about Sexual Coercion. *Annual Review of Critical Psychology*, 15: 26–49. ISSN 1746–739X

Sheehy, C. and Nayak, S. (2020) Black Feminist Methods of Activism Are the Tool for Global Social Justice and Peace. *Critical Social Policy*, 40(2): 234–257. https://doi.org/10.1177/0261018319896231

Soreanu, R. (2018) The Psychic Life of Fragments: Splitting from Ferenczi to Klein. *American Journal of Psychoanalysis*, 78(4): 421–444. https://doi.org/10.1057/s11231-018-9167-0

Tucker, S. (2011) Psychotherapy Groups for Traumatized Refugees and Asylum Seekers. *Group Analysis*, 44(1): 68–82. https://doi.org/10.1177/0533316410390478

Volkan, V. D. (2003) The Re-Libidinalization of the Internal World of a Refugee Family. *Group Analysis*, 36(4): 555–570. https://doi.org/10.1177/0533316403364012

Walshe, J. (2006) The Intermediate Space: The Border Country. *Group Analysis*, 39(2): 185–197.

Weinberg, H. (2007) So What Is This Social Unconscious Anyway? *Group Analysis*, 40(3): 307–322. https://doi.org/10.1177/0533316407076114

Winnicott, D. W. (1990 [1965]) *The Maturational Processes and the Facilitating Environment: Studies in the Theory of Emotional Development*. London: Karnac Books.

Yoa'd Ghanadry-Hakim (2020) *Palestine Counseling Centre (Beit Hanina branch) Café Palestine 4 30th May 2020 via UK-Palestine Mental Health Network (UKPMHN)*. http://psychicrefuge.com/en-research/palestine-mental-health [Accessed online 25th April 2022].

Yuval-Davis, N. (2006) 'Intersectionality and Feminist Politics.' Special Issue on 'Intersectionality'. *European Journal of Women's Studies*, 13: 193–209.

Chapter 6

Diffraction as the Group-Specific Phenomenon

Alasdair Forrest

Foulkes developed an original view of human life and psychopathology by look-ing at the world, and his patients, through a unique combination of lenses from other disciplines. In doing so, he integrated ideas from network theory, Gestalt psychology and neurology, and sociology with those of psychoanalysis. These ideas refined those from classic psychoanalysis, with its emphasis on drives, at a time when classic psychoanalysis was also being re-examined from the perspec-tive of Melanie Klein's ideas. Foulkes made new conceptualisations, at the level of interpersonal interaction in groups, of ideas that were core to psychoanalysis and thought of mainly in intrapsychic terms.

Klein's ideas derived from clinical observations of children and what she knew, largely through others, of patients with psychotic disorders. They did not come from other fields in the same way that Foulkes's did – or, of course, from his experience with groups. Foulkes's ideas have had less influence beyond their immediate field. That Klein's have had the influence they have demonstrates the enduring appeal to clinicians of clinical experience over theoretical frameworks. This is appropriate enough, given that psychotherapy is a clinical discipline whose theoretical frame-works are taken up or discarded insofar as they are helpful to the patient.

Applying an intersectional lens to group-analytic work, therefore, requires a clinically-oriented understanding of the ideas and how they interact with those already in currency in the group-analytic discourse and a willingness to be open to these ideas and to change (Nayak, 2021). This is an important invitation, which was extended to the field, not with an RSVP – *répondez, s'il vous plaît* – but instead with an urgency that goes beyond "if you please": group analysis needs outsider concepts, including intersectionality. The invitation should be taken up.

Just as Foulkes was willing to re-examine key principles from psychoanalysis, so group analysts now need to be willing to re-examine central ideas if they are to live in a way that serves our patients. Recently, the group-analytic literature has been engaging with different ideas around power, position, and privilege (e.g., Kent, 2021; Kinouani, 2020; Stevenson, 2020). This comes after a period of inter-est in the social unconscious. Basic ideas about group dynamics, such as Foulkes's group-specific factors of resonance, mirroring, translation, and condensation, have not been developed greatly in the last decades in spite of further clinical experience.

DOI: 10.4324/9781003232216-7

They could be developed, as Foulkes developed his idea, by bringing them into close communication with newer ideas in the context of clinical work.

Feminist writers have been developing the idea of diffraction since its introduction by Barad and development by Haraway. This intersectional idea develops the traditional idea of establishing knowledge through reflection, instead looking at how knowledge, positions, and ways of relating are constituted by intersecting waves of similarity and discrimination – but must always refer to material reality. There is an obvious connection with the Foulkesian concept of mirroring – and also with the idea of resonance. In this chapter, the concept of mirroring is reviewed, then the concept of diffraction is introduced. Following this, the concept is developed and used to illuminate clinical material.

Mirroring

Foulkes wrote on mirror reactions from his 1948 book onward (Foulkes, 1948). This is at a similar time to when his fellow member of the British Psychoanalytical Society, Melanie Klein, wrote on projective identification – first in passing (Klein, 1946). This was a time when British psychoanalysis was grappling with the more complex aspects of projection and non-verbal interpersonal emotional communication. Foulkes favoured concepts that linked to the group directly rather than to a repackaging of individual psychoanalytical concepts for the group and took little interest in projective identification, making only a passing reference to it.

If Klein took projection as her starting point, Foulkes took introjection as his. His writing about patients was not divorced from the material reality of their lives and what they had brought into their ways of relating to it – including the material conditions of the early post-War period.

In the initial exposition, he groups a larger number of ideas in the mirror reaction, including the fact that group members watch interactions between other group members. He seems at first to have it almost in an educative, spectator role – at least in part. He always saw it as a combination of processes, though. Earlier in the book, he recognises the two-dimensional nature of the mirror when he writes, from the position of the analyst in the group, of the patients, "they show us our own weaknesses in a mirror, like a caricature" (Foulkes, 1948:28). Yet, something more nuanced is in his writing from the beginning, such as when he writes "forces of identification and contrast are at work here" (Foulkes, 1948:167). From the beginning, he can therefore see that mirroring processes involve not just recognition and a sense of closeness but also rejection of what is seen. By the time of *Therapeutic Group Analysis*, he writes in a way that takes the concept away from any idea that is about learning by seeing and looks wholly to psychodynamics: "A person sees himself, or part of himself – often repressed parts of himself – reflected in the interactions of other group members" (Foulkes, 1964:110). He says that "this can be dissected into a number of psycho-analytic concepts, e.g., projection, identification, etc., but there are good grounds for putting these together and giving them a collective name, emphasising the 'mirror' part" (Foulkes, 1964:81).

Group analysts have since tended to see Foulkes as idealising of groups, ignoring the many comments of his wariness and these early statements that mirror reactions were not necessarily cosy moments of recognition.

The mirror reaction was then an important part of group-analytic thinking through Foulkes's life and in the period after his death. Pines reviewed and developed the concept, particularly in his Foulkes Lecture (Pines, 1982). He distinguished two forms of mirroring: one that was "primitive confrontation, direct and unreflective" (supp p. 16) and another "exploratory, negotiable and dialogical, between two or more persons who are sharing the same psychological space, one in which different points of view on the same experience can be explored. No mediation is needed" (supp p. 16–17). Like Zinkin (1983), a year later, he divided the concept in two between a kind of unbearable-seeing-with-rejection and a connected-seeing-with-recognition. The unbearable-seeing-with-rejection is the process of escalating, uncontained communication where two members reject what they cannot bear to see of themselves in the other person, which he called malignant mirroring.

Weinberg and Toder (2004) provide the most recent review of the concept of mirroring in the group-analytic literature. They describe things that are not relevant to this chapter but also divide mirror reactions into different forms, again recognising the distinction between alienating and recognition-creating mirroring.

All of these formulations, though, hint at a two-position process of reflected and reflector. It is not certain how this metaphor extends usefully to a group. Foulkes and Anthony (1957), attempting early on to resolve this perhaps, refer to the group as a "hall of mirrors" where an individual sees various aspects of themselves and can, over time, distinguish between what represents them and what does not, and can reconcile internal and external views of them. If, as group analysts, we rely on this two-person view of mirroring, we are at risk of falling into traps about pairs that exclude a broader conceptualisation of what is happening in the group.

This was the case in a closed group in which I was the conductor:

> *Increasingly obvious tit-for-tat hostility in a group came to the fore when one member of the pair wasn't there. "I can't be in this group with her. It's her or me".*

The second member never returned. What I had considered as a form of malignant mirroring left me feeling powerless to intervene with a process that somehow seemed to be between the two of them. Later, I shall describe a similar situation where recognition of points of similarity and difference across a group using a more diffractive perspective helped promote exchange rather than foster its rejection.

Mirroring, at least in some forms, is the truly chaotic form of recognition in groups. The affect is about surprise, and that may be alienating. Perhaps it is more alienating when someone's identity is characterised by feeling alienated – by abjection – because of the position in which there are placed by virtue of the colour of their skin (Hook, 2004) or where they have been made to internalise unconscious feelings of inferiority (as in the epidermalisation described by Fanon, 1952).

In my experience, most of the time, people in groups are not seeing themselves in others with complete recognition. More often, they see shades or hints, often on the edge of their awareness.

I think mirroring, split as it so often is, leads to an over-emphasis on benign mirror reactions when they may not be present. Pseudo-identifications are common early in the experience of the group as members find their feet with each other. Indeed, there were pseudo-identifications quite commonly in this new group – a lot of "that's exactly what is happening to me". In this closed group, which ran for six months, members spent the first four months being exactly the same as each other, likely to manage the anxiety generated by the time boundary. The last few months featured growing hostility and the departure described, which came with a renewed sense of solidarity-relief that this member had gone and very little progress after that.

However, some such superficial pseudo-identifications should probably not be dismissed. It may be better to recognise them as diffractive participation of a certain kind where there are points of similarity that look bright because they are newly-seen – as will be described in what follows. However, I was, too, reassured by them in the initial period of the group.

Diffraction

Barad has advanced the idea of diffraction as part of a complex of ideas that relies on the concept of intra-action. This is a term that seems, by its nature, group-analytic. Barad prefers the term to interaction since it does not rely on the idea of two separate bodies interacting as though they exist outside interaction, as pre-established actors. Instead, it suggests a process of resonance between them – and of transpersonal processes – such that the two are constituted in their intra-action. Foulkes wrote of transpersonal processes as being like X-rays passing through people. This is of his time. X-rays were relatively new in clinical usage by the time he was training as a doctor – and held a lot of promise. X-rays can diffract but do not in their diagnostic usage. In humans, they pass through bodies to different degrees depending on the constitution of the body part. Some, like bone, are relatively radio-opaque, so X-rays do not pass through them readily. They do not discolour the film behind. Others, like air, are radio-lucent, so X-rays do pass through them. The X-ray is monochrome because it is really only about density. Nothing of movement or angles is shown. The X-ray metaphor constrains our thinking, while one around diffraction can open it up – particularly as we consider how people are constituted by intra-action and by their differences.

Barad trained as a physicist, and the complex of ideas relies on the flexibility and surprises that come from the different views of matter developed in quantum physics. Group analysis has a history of taking an interest in this work (Dick, 1993). Of course, this is only by analogy – the very nature of quantum physics seems to be in recognising that what happens at one level (the subatomic) is different than what happens at another (the atomic). This is the same as how group analysts must remember that different concepts are needed in individual-level, small-group-level, large-group, and social formulations, since there is no particular reason why these should be the same.

Barad uses the two-slit or double-slit experiment as a foundation of their thought. This is an experimental design that they describe in two parts. First, one should imagine a light source behind a screen with two slits projecting onto another slit. Because the light is a wave, the new two waves, created by the slit, interfere with each other, producing a pattern that indicates that these are waves. Interestingly, electrons – so particles, not waves – do not behave as one may expect if one were to think they were particles like tennis balls being fired by a ball gun towards the device. They hit the screen with a probabilistic, diffraction-like pattern. Second, though, Barad describes an experiment in which there is a detector able to tell which slit a single electron is going through. If this detection experiment is at work, the electron does not behave like a wave but instead like a particle. There is an effect changed by the observation. She takes her thinking quite broadly into a set of ideas she describes as agential realism, which will not be discussed in detail here, but which basically places humans as actors in the universe alongside non-human objects, where there is a continuous process of interaction producing phenomena that become somehow intelligible even to non-humans, and are responded to (Pinch, 2011).

Barad's formulations have been criticised by physicists. The fundamental empirical basis they use to describe the idea of diffraction, the two-slit experiment, may not work as they describe it. In fact, not only does their interpretation come from only one view on quantum mechanics, but it is also argued by some to be highly eccentric and based on misunderstandings (Faye and Jaksland, 2021). Barad does not see quantum mechanics as an interesting perspective that can metaphorically assist us in understanding meaning – instead, seeing it as empirically true. Barad describes their view on diffraction in a way that makes it about the immanent nature of co-constituted actors who cannot exist outside of their interaction, much in the way Foulkes wrote about how an individual "can only artificially be considered in isolation, like a fish out of water" (1948:14–15). They write:

> *The key is understanding that identity is not essence, fixity or givenness, but a contingent iterative performativity, thereby reworking this alleged conflict into an understanding of difference not as an absolute boundary between object and subject, here and there, this and that, but rather as the effects of enacted cuts **in a radical reworking of cause and effect** .*
>
> (Barad, 2014:173–174; emphasis in original)

It is for physicists, not psychotherapists, to think about whether cause and effect can radically be reworked in terms of non-sentient entities. It may be that the language used here is confusing and leads to confusion in a kind of pathetic fallacy, where human elements are imputed because they are the only language possible. However, a radical reworking of cause and effect and a troubling of the absolute boundaries between subject and object are possible agents of change in human relations, such as in therapy groups. They also have broader applications in the social sphere. The difference is that Foulkes was not speaking literally when he spoke of a fish out of water – not in every aspect. In the same book, he finished by writing: "A good group, however, breeds and develops, creates and cherishes that most precious product: *the human individual*" (Foulkes, 1948:170; emphasis in original).

However they are taken, Barad's ideas have been influential in a trend in feminism known as the New Materialism. This is a broad idea that originated in feminist science studies. There, once simple metrics around publishing rates and the presence of, or exclusion of, women from disciplines were examined, the masculinist hegemony in the development of ideas was recognised and critiqued. Intersectional feminism, though, as originally articulated by Crenshaw, was far more obviously materialist – starting with Crenshaw's references to differential pay rates for Black women compared with White women and men and the difficulties Black women had in organising as a class in lawsuits, in the paper in which she introduced the term intersectionality (Crenshaw, 1989). There is no intersectionality that is not grounded completely in material reality, including money and poverty and the reality of bodies and their use and abuse. Notably, returning to Fanon (1952), he described the internalisation or epidermalisation of inferiority as part of a process only, alongside the economic aspect of difference. It has further resonances with group analysis because it yokes together the way power structures position people with empirical and biological facts. This is the clearest connection with Foulkesian psychology since Foulkes regarded the foundation matrix as linked to the material reality of the human species. Leaders in the feminist New Materialism, like Donna Haraway, use Barad's ideas in a more metaphorical way in aid of a project that questions the development of knowledge in the context of the marginalisation of women, poorer people, and people of colour, while not descending into a reality-denying relativism where the discourse is the only thing at hand. Haraway is not so grounded in quantum physics, but that does not stop her from grounding the ideas from Barad in bodies on the one hand and knowledge-production on the other.

> *So, I think my problem, and "our" problem, is how to have simultaneously an account of radical historical contingency for all knowledge claims and knowing subjects, a critical practice for recognizing our own "semiotic technologies" for making meanings, and a no-nonsense commitment to faithful accounts of a "real" world, one that can be partially shared and that is friendly to earthwide projects of finite freedom, adequate material abundance, modest meaning in suffering, and limited happiness.*

(Haraway, 1988:579)

Haraway's Critique of Reflexivity

Donna Haraway has, in particular, used Barad's idea of diffraction to re-examine the idea of reflection in various works. She has done this in a way that is relevant to clinical work in group analysis. Her thoughts are reviewed clearly and systematically by Campbell (2004).

Haraway uses reflexivity in its most nuanced and developed sense and still finds it lacking as an idea. She defines reflexivity not just in terms of the obvious consideration of what is happening with another but also considering one's own position and how it developed.

Reflection is, by its nature, a concept that is about two dimensions. The intersectional idea is that there are always far more than two dimensions. Moreover, Haraway proposes that reflection merely reproduces the same situation in a way that treats the other person not as an acting agent but instead as an object. It does not allow the "effects of connection, of embodiment, and of responsibility for an imagined elsewhere" (Haraway, cited in Campbell, 2004) but instead is narcissistic in quality and unlikely to unsettle a sense of position and power. Haraway argues that an enlivening, more genuine interaction relies not on representation and the idea of seeing oneself in others. It relies instead on what she calls a process of articulation or of creating relationships between actors to explore and develop an understanding based on differences. In this, she includes non-human actors, including objects of study in the natural sciences. She joins the material and the meaning-making by referring to "material-semiotic bodies". Poetically, she says that, like poems, "bodies as objects of knowledge are material-semiotic generative nodes" (Haraway, 1988).

By this, she means that there is no such thing as an object in our encountering of it without a social definition of where it begins and ends in a way that makes it what it is. This is not a solely social definition because it is largely informed by what is materially evident, but the world of meaning and the world of matter are the same one. Group analysis can become ridiculous if Foulkes's misquoted idea that there is no such thing as an individual is taken too literally. Bodies, though, and in this context, human bodies, are constituted in the manner of their social encounter by meaning-making processes and, of course, also generate meaning. In another meaning-making way, these bodies – which are who we are and not objects – are racialised, gendered, and marked by trauma or advantage or both, and more. However, if a patient in a group is seen in the light of one or more essentialised identity characteristics alone, then they are turned into an object rather than seen as the material-semiotic generative node they are. They are constituted by but also active contributors to meaning-making.

"Racist social structures create racist psychic structures" (Oliver, 2001:34). What, then, is the role of reflection? How does that allow any movement from a position that is always-already constituted and always-already defined by racist, homophobic, and misogynistic ways of being and being-made-to-be? There is limited ability to make headway in untangling the pain of oppression if one can only see bits of oneself in others, or not see them, or reluctantly see them with disavowal. How does a Black man, trying to make sense of his experience of the world, come to terms with the fact that the person most imbued with racist hatred of blackness was a parent who was White if there are no moving parts alive in the group for him to find some points of recognition, although different, and some points of difference, although recognisable? Mirroring and resonance need to find a way to be considered as one.

Diffraction as a Central Process in Groups

Having heard that a man had done something similar to what had been done to her, a group member said: "What you did is like what happened to me. But it's not exactly the same".

Groups create an alternative situation in which relationships can be re-attempted and, through this, change can take place inside and outside the group. In the moment in an established group, described previously, something that was not quite mirroring took place. Instead, it was a process of partial recognition and partial difference. This was the start of a long process of difficult but reparative work for both and for the group as a whole.

In the group, there was a full range of responses, immediate and delayed, to what was being discussed. As Foulkes (1964:290) said: "Resonance is intended to denote the fact that not only is there an unconscious communication between individuals but also that this unconscious communication is highly selective and specific". Such an interaction is hard to capture in full view and living experience on the page.

One member said he was brave to have said what he said. Another said they feared for him. Another said they didn't know what to say and were now scared of him. Another said she had been through something similar to the woman.

Which were the mirror reactions, and which were the resonances? I believe that the group-analytic literature is less explicitly centred on group-dynamic phenomena in recent years than it was early in the discipline's history. The focus has often moved to the social unconscious. With the idea of the mirror reaction, the division between more benign and malignant forms of it may have retarded the development of the idea. Just as resonance does not refer solely to times when there is an agreement of experience ("that resonates with me") but instead relates to the sum-total of emotional reactions to what is going on in the group, so mirroring has been limited by its current exposition. Diffraction provides an alternative. Altering Foulkes's words: this can be dissected into a number of group-analytic concepts, e.g., mirror reaction, resonance, etc., but there are good grounds for putting these together and giving them a collective name: diffractive processes.

Instead of seeing interaction in a group as being in a hall of mirrors, we could see the group as a collection of prisms. Light coming straight towards the prism's edge could be reflected, perhaps at times pass right through. It may miss the prism entirely. At other times – indeed almost all the time – instead, it hits the prism at an angle, and the light is split. Some are seen with recognition; some are not; much passes on to other prisms. The different parts of the spectrum that appear more or less around each prism will vary from one to another – and be more or less similar or more or less different from the others. I think this is a helpful way of thinking about the group. It takes some of the nature of the mirror reaction – the seeing with recognition and the seeing with rejection – while also allowing for surprising points of similarity and difference, shared and not shared in different measures, in a way that recalls resonance.

In time, the group has come to hear about the experience of growing up in poverty and how that differs across countries and racialised identities in a way that leaves the women who experienced it with differences, as well as with similarities. Some things will be understood, and some will not. The group has also come to hear the differences in how to be a man, and a professional man, and a man in front of other men, and a man with women in front of powerful men. A whole range of reactions and counter-reactions have emerged from a developing capacity to imagine oneself in the other's position – sort of.

Diffraction Makes the Central Process an Intersectional Process – With Questionable Opportunities for the Conductor

Analytical categories like "race", "gender", "class" and the hegemonic practices associated with them (racism, sexism, classism to which imperialism and homophobia certainly could be added) are mutually constitutive, not conceptually distinct.

(Hancock, 2016:71)

Hancock defines intersectionality in the tightest of ways: she says one cannot talk about oppressed positions of power and privilege in terms only of one essentialised identity category. In the group interaction described previously, what starts off as a discussion of an interaction – with all the involvement of being an actor, seeing other actors act, and acting back with them – soon enough becomes about how one learned to act that way. Soon enough after that, it becomes about who one is and how one came to be enabled and constrained.

Diffraction goes further than mirroring and resonance can because it allows the experience to be anchored in intersectional experiences of power, position, and privilege. Rather than the individual being a nodal point in a network, they can be seen as constituted by the intersection of different waves both outside the group (what Foulkes called by the rarely-used word plexus) and inside the group.

If, as Seshadri-Crooks (2000) argues, whiteness is the socially default state that forms other racial subjectivities in opposition to itself, a mirror-reaction kind of reflection would oppose any sense of a more nuanced connection that accepts the gaps between racialised experiences but also finds points of connection. The work of understanding, and of therapy, could come from articulating points of similarity, including surprising ones, in the kind of solidarity-making work that intersectionality suggests between people with differences of power, position, and privilege – rather than defining them by identity characteristics alone.

But these identity characteristics do not lose a material-semiotic reality just by being interrogated. Group analysts working in communities where, for example, more than 90% of the population is racialised as White face an ethical challenge in their conducting. They are facing an empty category, Whiteness, that is anything but empty. They may consider racialised and racist aspects of relating to be alive in the life and interactions of the group as that default state that resists consideration by being the blank category. Do they interpret this, thereby seeming to introduce into the group something that was not in the material brought by the patients? Does failing to do this not reproduce racism in the most obvious way? Equally, does doing so merely pay lip service – producing an imaginary, objectifying reflexive show without an engagement with an immediate, material-semiotic encounter that finds points of difference and similarity? But does offering space in a group to a Black woman, say, or two, or three, to take up that side of the interaction constitute therapy or work on behalf of the whole group that replicates the racist dynamic? These are problems of conducting that lead group analysts naturally into a space of two-dimensional relating – including with the imagined other that is so different by being only imagined.

There is no intersectionality without race in a racist society. It may be, though, that an intersectional focus on differences in power, privilege, and position that can come about from the broader focus on diffractive processes allows members of the group to articulate their difference in a way that permits, and indeed welcomes, an understanding of the differences not recognised. Trying to work with this framework in mind is difficult because the tendency around painful difference is to constrain rather than enable discourse, and the conductor can easily be drawn into this.

An Asian man joined an established group, being the only member of the group who was not White. Nine months in, after he had made some comments about himself that were spoken over, for the second time, I said that I thought there was ignoring of any idea that his background or experience was any different from anyone else in the group, and that this may come about from fear of everyone hurting each other. This was again disavowed, while later, several members of the group expressed annoyance at my actions in various other things that had not been of concern before.

In this situation, again, I think I failed to recognise the need to place in the foreground the possibility of points of connection as well as points of difference and repeated a kind of singling-out on the one hand that was avoided by stronger disavowal on the other. Yet again, I fell into a kind of trap of repeating a racist dynamic.

Conductors have long recognised that the stance they take can need to be modified to work with a particular dynamic. I have come to believe that, with these oppressive dynamics around racism, misogyny, homophobia, and others, a simply interpretive focus is not sufficient. Instead, although it risks a more directive stance at times – which always has the possibility of the conductor steering the material in a way that is more driver than conductor – I have started to reflect on links between people with differences in identity characteristics but akin experiences of injustice. For example:

> *In a group where a member had grown up with very little resources, material or otherwise, and seemed to find it hard to make connections with other members, I said that I turned to another member and said that I knew some of his story, and that I could hear similarities alongside the obvious major differences, and wondered if he could. This did promote a connection that later on became, naturally, a stronger connection as it developed without such explicit linking from me.*

I am not settled in my mind about this course of action. My guide is the idea of diffraction – and that intersectional differences push people apart such that they may need the conductor's steer to see initial points of connection – and that, in particular, racist and misogynistic social and psychic structures mean that it is not always possible simply to trust the group to sort these things out, at least not initially.

Conclusion

In attempting to respond to Nayak's (2021) invitation to bring outsider concepts into group analysis, and vice versa, a reworking of the mirror reaction and resonance is proposed. This recognises the interdependence of these two phenomena and seeks to ground them in an intersectional understanding of the positions in which people are placed by interacting social forces.

Just as Foulkes thought there to be good grounds for bringing together several psychoanalytic concepts, I believe there are good grounds for bringing together resonance and mirroring and considering them as diffraction. With this slight change in emphasis, I have slightly changed my conducting to recognise better that power, privilege, and position are alive in our groups and that we are not yet, as group analysts, where we should or could be in developing our clinical tools for working with them. If we can refine what we are doing, we should be able to better use our groups to serve our patients who come to them looking for help. In all their difference, we may be able to cherish that most precious product: *the human individual.*

References

Barad, K. (2014) Diffracting Diffraction: Cutting Together-Apart. *Parallax*, 20: 168–187.
Campbell, K. (2004) The Promise of Feminist Reflexivities: Developing Donna Haraway's Project for Feminist Science Studies. *Hypatia*, 19(1): 162–182. www.jstor.org/stable/3810936
Crenshaw, K. (1989) Demarginalizing the Intersection of Race and Sex: A Black Feminist Critique of Antidiscrimination Doctrine. *University of Chicago Legal Forum*, 1989: 139–168.
Dick, B. (1993) The Group Matrix as a Holomovement and Quantum Field. *Group Analysis*, 26(4): 469–480.

Fanon, F. (1952). *Black Skin, White Masks*. Paris: Editions Seuil.

Faye, J. and Jaksland, R. (2021) Barad, Bohr, and Quantum Mechanics. *Synthese*, 199: 8231–8255.

Foulkes, S. H. (1948) *Introduction to Group Analytic Psychotherapy*. London: Karnac.

Foulkes, S. H. (1964) *Therapeutic Group Analysis*. London: Allen and Unwin [Reprinted London: Karnac].

Foulkes, S. H. and Anthony, J. (1957) *Group Psychotherapy: The Psychoanalytic Approach*. London: Karnac.

Hancock, A.-M. (2016) *Intersectionality: An Intellectual History*. Oxford: Oxford University Press.

Haraway, D. (1988) Situated Knowledges: The Science Question in Feminism and the Privilege of Partial Perspective. *Feminist Studies*, 14(3): 575–599.

Hook, D. (2004) Racism as Abjection: A Psychoanalytic Conceptualisation for a Post-Apartheid South Africa. *South African Journal of Psychology*, 34(4): 672–703.

Kent, J. (2021) Scapegoating and the 'Angry Black Woman'. *Group Analysis*, 54(3): 354–371.

Kinouani, G. (2020) Difference, Whiteness and the Group Analytic Matrix: An Integrated Formulation. *Group Analysis*, 53(1): 60–74.

Klein, M. (1946) Notes on Some Schizoid Mechanisms. *The International Journal of Psychoanalysis*, 27: 99–110.

Nayak, S. (2021) Black Feminist Intersectionality Is Vital to Group Analysis: Can Group Analysis Allow Outsider Ideas In? *Group Analysis*, 54(3): 337–353.

Oliver, K. (2001) *Witnessing: Beyond Recognition*. Minneapolis: University of Minnesota Press.

Pinch, T. (2011) Karen Barad, Quantum Mechanics, and the Paradox of Mutual Exclusivity [Review of *Meeting the Universe Halfway: Quantum Physics and the Entanglement of Matter and Meaning*, by K. Barad]. *Social Studies of Science*, 41(3): 431–441.

Pines, M. (1982) 6th S. H. Foulkes Annual Lecture of the Group-Analytic Society. *Group Analysis*, 15(2): S1–S26.

Seshadri-Crooks, K. (2000) *Desiring Whiteness: A Lacanian Analysis of Race*. London: Routledge.

Stevenson, S. (2020) Psychodynamic Intersectionality and the Positionality of the Group Analyst: The Tension Between Analytical Neutrality and Inter-Subjectivity. *Group Analysis*, 53(4): 498–514.

Weinberg, H. and Toder, M. (2004) The Hall of Mirrors in Small, Large and Virtual Groups. *Group Analysis*, 37(4): 492–507.

Zinkin, L. (1983) Malignant Mirroring. *Group Analysis*, 16(2): 113–126.

Chapter 7

Missing Dialogues

Dick Blackwell and Claire Bacha

Dick Blackwell and Claire Bacha were members of a virtual online group organising a webinar to commemorate the September 2021 special issue of the journal *Group Analysis* on Racism (Borossa, 2021). *Group Analysis* is published by the Group Analytic Society International (GASi), a professional organisation for group analysts. The UK's main training organisation for group analysts, the Institute of Group Analysis (IGA), is a different body. Both authors have been concerned about the practice of the IGA. Bacha is involved in the Power, Position, and Privilege group (PPP) that seeks to examine and challenge the way in which group-analytic training excludes and marginalises minoritised and oppressed groups of people. Blackwell advocates for challenging the institutional racism and class prejudice of Group Analysis, and argues for its decolonisation. He argues that Group Analysis training should carry a "health warning" for Black and working-class students.

They are members of a group email server. On 6 September at 14:46, Blackwell suggested that authors might attend the Group Analytic Society (GASi) Journal Club when it discussed the special issue. A comment was made about one participant's previous experience with GASi, which left them unenthusiastic about further involvement.

On 7 September at 7:14, Bacha wrote that she heard the point being made but was uncomfortable with the rift.

Thus began the following correspondence between two experienced group analysts long involved in training. Small edits have been made for publication, but the spirit of the exchange is preserved. It shows opportunities and difficulties in applying intersectional ideas to group-analytic training and to the group-analytic corpus. Fundamentally, as it develops, the correspondents disagree on whether this constitutes a dialogue at all. Bacha suggests it does, while Blackwell feels that the points he has been making for years are not taken up, which defeats the prospect of dialogue. Both correspondents claim that the other is missing them, or that they are missing something, or being missed.

Most of the book deals with elements of intersectionality in the foundation matrix – what is held in common in society as a whole. Group Analysts, though, increasingly think in terms of a tripartite matrix (Hopper, 2018). This chapter addresses the dynamic matrix. It is right that intersectional experience is considered in the dynamic

DOI: 10.4324/9781003232216-8

matrix of the key organisation involved in group-analytic training, the Institute of Group Analysis in London, and in the membership organisation, the Group Analytic Society International. If Group Analysts truly believe that individuals are social to their core, it is important to track and be alive in these movements in the dynamic matrix. The potential and difficulty in doing so is exemplified here.

From: Dick Blackwell
Date: 7 September 2021, 18:56

To: All

It is important to recognise that GASi is not a unity. It's an arena of struggle. Boycotting GASi because of how its Management Committee operates is like boycotting the IGA because of its Board and leaving PPP (the Power, Position, and Privilege group in the IGA) to fight its struggle alone. A Management Committee can do some dumb-ass things, and those of us fighting racism need them to be challenged. But ignoring them doesn't help us. It helps them.

To fight racism and colonialism, we need international solidarity and links between the progressive tendencies in different organisations like GASi and the IGA. In the wider world of psychotherapy, it's starting to look like there's a case for links and mutual support between the progressive elements in different psychotherapy institutes. That's the only way I can see that we're going to decolonise psychotherapy in the UK. And until that happens, the institutional racism in virtually all the trainings is going to continue.

Bw,
Dick

From: Claire Bacha
Date: 8 September 2021, 10:00
To: Dick Blackwell

Hi Dick,

Could it be that seeing GASi as an arena of struggle is part of the problem? We don't want to struggle with each other. We want to dialogue as group analysts. I don't see the struggle approach as being fruitful of anything except more splits, polarizations and factions. When there are splits, polarizations and factions, people stop talking to each other openly.

Also, when I hear about decolonization, all I can think of is that we are all colonized by Neoliberal capitalism, which turns us against each other. In that case, we all need to decolonize and also to become something else, as yet unknown. Is this what you mean? Am I missing something?

Bw,
Claire

Afterthought: Elias might say that we are always becoming something else, as yet unknown.

From: Dick Blackwell
Date: 9 September 2021, 16:47
To: Claire Bacha

Hi Claire,

You are missing so much, it's difficult to know where to begin. 500 years of history? (Since Columbus). 400 years of history? (Slavery and the struggle against it). 300 years of history? (The class struggle that produced the Welfare State and the NHS? They weren't gifts from the ruling class or the petit bourgeoisie). Do you imagine that an organisation is somehow immune to all these struggles and not determined and permeated by them? Then there's 100 years of history of Foulkes and GA (since his time in the Frankfurt Institute's building) and the history of GAS members struggling to de-centre London to make GAS 'European'; and the little 'i' in GASi to reflect the compromise between those who want a genuinely international society and those terrified of losing their white European home. Not to mention the colonising of students' minds by some current IGA trainings.

Farhad and I have been writing about this stuff for almost 30 years (Blackwell, 1994; Dalal, 1993). We and our work have been 'negated' in much the way I described 'negation' as a central feature of colonialism in my Foulkes lecture in 2003 (Blackwell, 2003)! We've been struggling for that length of time to be heard. To even get these issues on the agenda, whether or not anyone agrees with us. Our books and papers are systematically excluded from a lot of reading lists, so the debates never happen. Large groups of the last 18 months have featured a systematic negation and erasure of black and working-class voices no matter how often attention is drawn to this exclusion. An online symposium disabled 'Chat' in the large group in order, according to one insider, to shut me up and block the link-ups being made in 'Chat' between black and other marginalised members that the mainstream prefers to ignore/negate.

In the wider world of psychoanalysis and psychoanalytic psychotherapy, some of us have spent decades challenging a status quo in which black analysands routinely have their experiences of racism denied and reassigned to something else by their analysts. Most Black psychotherapy students have a painful and alienating experience, as do those who've tried to pioneer something different: Jaffa Kareem, Lennox Thomas, Fakhry Davids, etc. I expect the Black women pioneers I'm not in touch with suffer something similar. Black students coming to train these days need to be given a health warning: 'This training can do you damage!' Working class students and members of other marginalized groups suffer similarly, though maybe not quite as badly. None of this is secret. It's just covered up.

I thought the habitual denial of racism in the analytic situation was improving, but my colleague Guilaine Kinouani (2020b) assures me that it isn't.

Yes, we're colonized by Neoliberal capitalism. But in every colonial situation, we find those who resist, those who succumb, those who compromise, those who feather their own nests and those who get into bed with the coloniser. So, who's? I pointed out nearly 20 years ago that group analytic language was being colonised. Farhad Dalal (2015) has repeatedly pointed out the adoption and penetration of 'New Public Management' in IGA London. It can only happen with Group Analysis's cooperation/capitulation/complicity. So, who takes responsibility for that?

There is right now a struggle in the IGA training faculty about whether the term 'decolonising' can be used. It's amazing! All over the world, academics are talking and writing about decolonising the European-based academy, but GA seems to want to remain oblivious to it. Erica Burman (2021) gives a keynote at the Symposium about Fanon, and still, GA remains oblivious. I've then heard in GASi how welcome Fanon is, and what a pity we've not heard of him before. Really? Could it be we've been stubbornly resisting knowing about him? Or working hard to forget what we've already heard?

Three years ago, a proposal for a seminar on 'racism, class, gender and marginalization' was rejected by the IGA board, who not only refused to support it but also blocked our use of the building on the 50th Anniversary of May '68, forcing us to hire another hall.

Your vision of this all changing through a 'dialogue' applying conventional group analytic concepts reads like a combination of GA omnipotence and white fragility. As if GA's institutional racism is like Sleeping Beauty's slumber, just waiting for Prince Charming's kiss to break the spell. Your anxiety about 'splits, polarizations and factions' sounds like an endorsement of Kehinde Andrews' thesis that 'whiteness is a psychosis' (Andrews, 2018:193–201). Maybe a breakdown is long overdue.

Re: your mention of Elias: It's unclear how many other sociologists get quoted in GA. But Elias seems to have few rivals. Yet since he was writing, there have been a few developments: a new sociology of deviance (late 1960s) and of race and racism (same period), followed by post-colonial studies, subaltern studies, cultural studies, queer theory and of course feminism, almost all of which seem to have passed GA by. Mainstream GA remains rooted in the 1950s. I don't think that's inertia. It's resistance! The maintenance and defence of a white, Western, middle-class, professional, heteronormative, patriarchal ghetto.

What your response reminds me of is the terror (and it's not just anxiety but terror and panic) within so much of GA about any sort of serious conflict, especially political conflict. When you talk about containing conflict, I hear damping it down and glossing it over, avoiding recognising its depth and its true nature. Civilising it for those who don't feel too harmed and dehumanised by it. That is, to a large extent, why feminism has made so few real inroads into GA. A serious dialogue about patriarchy is far too dangerous. We might fall out. The routine personal politicking and back-stabbing that's been endemic in GA's internal dynamics might get exposed. And we don't go near the fact that until Suryia Nayak came along, it's been a notably white, middle-class, heter-onormative feminism knocking politely at the patriarchal door. When we get black contributions to a workshop on 'Internalised Misogyny', for example, they're promptly erased from the subsequent discussion.

What you've suggested here about there not really being a struggle except in my mind and not being able to engage with the idea of 'decolonization', is, in effect, adding another brick to what Guilaine (Kinouani, 2020a) and I (Blackwell, 2020) have both called 'the impenetrable wall of whiteness' and an additional piece of white glass to what Anne here has so eloquently described as the 'white mirror' (Aiyegbusi, 2021a). It's also reminiscent of David Cameron declaring a class war called 'austerity' then telling us 'We're all in it together!' The struggle is right here.

Bw,
Dick

From: Claire Bacha
Date: 10 September 2021, 12:43
To: Dick Blackwell

Dear Dick,

I am not discounting history, far from it. I am hoping that you will be able to help me understand better the links between anticolonialism and anticapitalism and how these links help to inform what we do next. In this respect, I have been reading Hannah Arendt and the points that she makes about where things start.

I would start with the history of capitalism, maybe with the Black Death in the 1300s, and look at the further development of capitalism into colonialism. I saw a piece recently that put the origins of our present world in 1492 when the Americas were discovered. I think that there is a difference between starting in 1300 and starting in 1492. I understand how capitalism created both wealth and poverty here and then in the rest of the world. I would not make them separate processes and struggles, would you?

I agree that we cannot isolate the IGA and GASi from the rest of the world. With the idea of what might make a group analytic organization, I have watched, like you, how we have gone from a more participatory and chaotic organization to one that is based on the prevailing neoliberalism of our time. Like you, I have been disturbed by this process and its effects on our training. However, I am mindful that I do not want to throw out what is valuable about group analysis with what it does not do. I think that group analysis holds a great potential for constructive change, and not only on a clinical level. I think that you must think so too, or you would not struggle so hard and so long with it. I doubt that the situation will improve until we offer something better to improve it. This is why I think that inclusivity in group analysis implies the need to change, and this change makes us stronger, bigger and wiser.

Thank you for clarifying part of the historical split between the IGA and GASi for me. I had not thought about the opening to Europe and the resistance to that as part of the split. I was part of the original group of students who challenged London-centrism from the North of England, meeting the same resistance. This resistance was difficult to understand at the time. It still is. I understand it as part of colonialism. What you said about IGA resistance to Europe helps me to understand the resistance to accepting Manchester as an equal partner in group analysis.

Basically, in Manchester, we adopted the European block model and put in enough hours to satisfy the IGA London requirements. It still took us ten years and a degree of political mobilization to gain full IGA membership. The Manchester Courses have not split from the IGA. The IGA is vastly different, and so is therapy in the rest of England, in some part, because of what we did, and do, in Manchester. We promoted a way of exporting the London trainings to the benefit of London and of the areas outside of London, too.

I take all your points about large groups. I can see the methods of the establishment of the elite. I can see people turning away from conflict and difference. I saw some of the dynamics between you and the larger group in the Internalised Misogyny Workshop. I thought that you should have been in the group and not taking potshots from the sidelines. It was distracting. You were encouraged to come into the group in the end. I have nothing against anger. It should be able to be in the group, contained, listened to, thought about and responded to. People are listening now more than they have been. History is important, but it is not everything.

I am sorry that you could not see what I was saying as new and different from 'GA omnipotence and white fragility'. I cannot actually see what I said to make you think this except to use the group analytic concepts that you are treating with contempt. I would never say that there is nothing else. However, I think that Group Analysis and Norbert Elias (1991) (and Hannah Arendt (1951, 1998) add something crucially important to the mix of anticapitalism and anticolonialism that we need to escape neoliberal capitalism and something else to be discovered.

This missing ingredient to get us to something else is the capacity to dialogue. Decolonizing the curriculum is an important part of this in the training. The real anger and hurt belong in our groups and in our institution, wherever they are created. Sometimes, breakdown is necessary, but mostly, breakdown happens when the feelings are not contained (different from damping down and glossing over), and it is the containment that we need to work on instead of the psychosis of turning away and splitting. I believe that we are doing some important part of this experiential work in PPP. This is what is new. You should come.

I did not say that the struggle was all in your mind. I was wondering if struggle just brings more struggle in GASi, as everywhere else. Not the same thing. Maybe it is time for you to try something else.

I think that you are angry, but not with me personally. You seem to have missed me completely, at least, I hope that you have. I don't think that you have answered my question about anticolonialism and anticapitalism. I sense that they are not the same, and I find this confusing.

Bw,
Claire

From: Dick Blackwell
Date: 16 September 2021, 17:07
To: Claire Bacha

Hi Claire,

I think capitalism only really got underway with the industrial revolution in Europe, which was built on cotton. Labour is the most variable cost of production, so cheap labour is vital for profits and consolidation. So European Industrialisation was built, essentially, on slavery in the cotton fields.

Hardly any struggles are separate. It's just different fronts in the same war. I stay in GA because of its roots in dialectics and democratic process/praxis. These days, I think more in terms of 'resistance' than 'constructive change' because we've been fighting a rear-guard for half a century, but I'm getting just a little more optimistic.

Just to be clear about 'decolonisation'. I have little interest in 'decolonising the curriculum' if that's all that's going to be decolonised. Putting Kimberlé Crenshaw, bell hooks and Angela Davis, and indeed Suryia Nayak and Anne Aiyegbusi, on a reading list doesn't go very far if they're going to be taught in the same authoritarian way and examined through dissertations marked by politburo panels of readers, who probably know less than the students. I start with Paulo Freire (1996) and Ivan Illich (1971). That begins to decolonise the structure and process of learning in GA.

I don't think I've treated any GA concepts with contempt. What I'm critical, if not contemptuous of, is mainstream GA's refusal to develop its thinking beyond a small cluster of concepts or to critically rethink them, particularly in the light of another 70 years of social and political theory. Foulkes, as Erica Burman said at the online symposium, is still revered (as the writer of the 'bible') rather than critiqued as a pre-1960s psychiatrist and psychoanalyst who was radical for his time, just like Freud. Their ideas have been reified by the positivist thinking inherent in the neoliberal project that has permeated GA, instrumentalising it as a technology of social control.

Two final points. We may not get rid of power, but we could share it more evenly and be more aware of its capacity to corrupt. Re: 'good authority': the only thing that can earn 'authority' the right to be considered as 'good' is its accountability to those over whom it is exercised, and its willingness to be challenged by them. Not many of those 'in authority' can currently meet those criteria. And the only alternatives to 'struggle' are submission or collaboration.

Bw,
Dick

From: Claire Bacha
Date: 26 September 2021, 8:31
To: Dick Blackwell

Dear Dick,

I think that it matters when we put the beginnings of things. I would argue that capitalism began in the 1300s with the beginning of the formation of the working class. It was the 'invention' of waged labour that created the capitalist relationship. It is this relationship, the separation of work from the means of production and the power relationship, that the separation entails, that defines capitalism. In this sense, capitalism created both wealth and poverty. Poverty created Industrialisation, and that started with wool, which came before cotton. It was an internal colonization first.

We cannot separate capitalism and colonialism, but they are not the same either. This matters because when you put capitalism as synonymous with Industrialisation in the 1850s, you put the emphasis on colonization as the way that primitive accumulation of capital created capitalism and globalization. This is undoubtedly true, but then you also take the emphasis off of the relationship of exploitation, which is at the heart of capitalist processes. This is important to us in Group Analysis because we are involved in understanding relationships, the traumas involved in relationships and how to heal them. We do this by facilitating external and internal dialogue.

The project of decolonizing by facilitating external and internal dialogue is deeply political. We must have a dialogue about how politically sensitive and important group analysis is. We are starting to do this. The decolonization of the curriculum is one important part of our communication with each other about who we are and where we come from, including the dialogues that we have with our students and our patients. Speaking and listening to each other. We need to revise our concepts and our techniques, and we do this in PPP. This is one way we can decolonize our minds from neoliberalism, which is at the heart of modern colonization. This process involves all of us.

I have written a response (2021) to one of Farhad's papers (Dalal, 2021) about the ethics of supervision (Bacha, 2021). I agree we need to be clear that we are practicing what we are teaching in our training and in our institution. Where do you think that the resistances to change reside? Perhaps we need to be more specific and think about how we have a response to neoliberalism that is more than resistance. You mentioned the dissertation. Is there something that is happening particularly there?

I would love to see you be more active in PPP. Have you thought about it?

Bw,
Claire

From: Dick Blackwell
Date: 3 October 2021, 19:34
To: Claire Bacha

Thanks, Claire. I'm aware that my version of history tends not to go back far beyond the Industrial Revolution, the Enlightenment and the French Revolution. I think the history of the formation and development of economic and relational patterns is important. Even though, in Morton's People's History (1989 [1938]), for example, while he likens 14th-century Yeomen Guilds to Trade Unions, he does not see the Trade Union movement as getting underway until the 18th century. That's when I think the dialectic of labour and capital takes shape, providing the context for the next 300 years of history that we're still living.

I don't think neoliberalism is part of a smooth and continuous development of capitalism, so much as a dialectical response to increasing democracy, trade unions and grassroots power post-WW2. The response must be to promote grassroots resistance, which is why the power structure of GA is important. Capitalism doesn't have to be exploitative if the workers have power within the organisation.

The resistances in GA are part of the permeation of GA by class conflicts through which middle-class racism develops and is refracted. I'm not sure all *our* minds are colonised by neo-liberalism (some of us have been resisting and fighting it from day one), but the IGA institutionally certainly is. The whole idea of marking student dissertations is an internalisation of the commodification of knowledge and the neoliberal creation of a top-down authority structure.

Inclusivity can only result from the demands and insistence of those who want to be included. Power is seldom, if ever, conceded without a struggle. That's where I think we are in GA.

I haven't joined PPP because the struggle needs to be fought on more than one front. Being a fellow traveller can be more advantageous than being a member, and there's an important military concept called 'crossfire'.

Bw,
Dick

From: Claire Bacha
5 October 2021, 8:04
To: Dick Blackwell

Dear Dick,

If you are interested in the early transition from feudalism to capitalism, there is a very good book called *Poverty and the State* (Novak, 1988). It clarified a lot for me about the origins of capitalism, the state and poverty, which are bound up with each other. Capitalism won't get any less exploitive or extractive any time soon. Possibly not before we destroy the planet. I don't think that capitalism can be made good. We need something else, and we need group analysis, or something similar, to bring that about.

I agree about grassroots response. Grassroots response is not just about activism and agitation, though. It also recognizes our own self- and group-enlightened interests and mandates a better kind of democracy. This is where group analysis comes in. We cannot think about grassroots resistance without also thinking about better dialogue, where conflicts and dialectics can actually be resolved. I don't think that uncontained conflict can lead anywhere except to having factions, war, violence and more violence. This is where racism is situated. We have the theory and the practice to begin to develop better and more widely accepted forms of dialogue. This is what we are doing in PPP and why it is important for you to join.

All our minds are colonized by neoliberalism. No one can exempt themselves from that, not even you. The danger of not being aware of the colonization is that we act on it. In actually-existing neoliberalism, it is alright to have a dialectic (conflict) between capital and labour as long as labour wins only little things. This is one of the aspects of the present moment that is so disturbing for me. The present attack is on the social and political processes of being held accountable.

As for racism arising out of colonialism, I invite you to read my paper with Sue Einhorn (Bacha et al., 2021) about antisemitism. Capitalism profoundly changed the nature of racism when making people into commodities, marked by race. I think that those ideas make sense. They make the point that racism and antisemitism are connected at their roots, historically.

I don't know anything about the problems around the dissertation. Do we need to look into it as PPP?

I was also interested in your use of the term 'crossfire'. I am not sure that I see the point of crossfire from a military point of view. Hearing things in stereo coming from different sources is very powerful, though. We know this from working in groups. I also found a lot of references to being 'caught in the crossfire' and how crossfire is dangerous to civilians and bystanders. We also know this from working in groups. There is a difference between an adversarial politics and a politics aimed at dialogue. We don't want to kill off the bystanders. I don't think that we want to kill off the perpetrators, either. Or do we? What kind of politics do we need to practice as group analysts to improve our understanding and effectiveness? Certainly, inclusivity is part of our politics: difficult but with constructive consequences, and it feels good.

Bw,
Claire

From: Dick Blackwell
Date: 7 October 2021, 17:29
To: Claire Bacha

If adversarial politics precluded dialogue, we wouldn't have the 'Good Friday Agreement' in Northern Ireland. The historic problem for GA is how to have a dialogue with the enemy, which is something trade unionists have known how to do for a long time. But middle-class psycho-professionals don't like learning from the proletariat. So, GA goes on being bad at it. I wrote about it so long ago (1980s) I've practically forgotten it (Blackwell, 1988). It's never been taken up.

There's a common narrative that slavery was defeated by Wilberforce. Toussaint Louverture and the armed struggle of the slaves are readily overlooked. Black History Month may be a good time to resurrect the real history. And the historical necessity of Malcolm X for Martin Luther King's voice to get heard.

Re: the dissertations, I think that if PPP is to generate far-reaching changes, it needs to look at the power structures of the trainings and the processes of marginalisation they produce.

Bw,
Dick

From: Claire Bacha
Date: 8 October 2021, 11:01
To: Dick Blackwell

Dear Dick,

I have nothing against adversarial politics. I understand that adversarial politics are necessary. My point about group analysis is that we are experts in group conversations. I agree that we should be better at what you are calling 'dialogue with the enemy'. Of course, we are not the only people who know about it. But we can add a lot to any understanding of dialogue. We have a good thing. We can make it better. My point about group analysis is that group analysis is not the enemy. We have the focus on interaction in groups that should be helpful in adversarial situations. If it is not, then we focus on what needs to be different or is missing. We are being told by our students and colleagues of colour that something important is missing. I am concerned about this. I don't think there is a simple answer, but there are ways forward.

Ireland is a good case in point. You could argue that the peace was also started by the women's civil rights movement and then won by the dialogues that took place between Martin McGuinness and the British in the back channels of a fish shop owner's home.

PPP is looking at the power processes and the processes of marginalization, both in the trainings and in the membership. That is what it is for.

Bw,
Claire

From: Dick Blackwell
Date: 13 October, 19:18
To: Claire Bacha

Dear Claire,

On Hannah Arendt and Norbert Elias: Arendt has been dead for 45 years. GA has hardly taken on board her ideas of the 'banality of evil', let alone participatory democracy. Elias has been dead for at least a quarter of a century and had little impact on GA until Farhad drew attention to him. GA is basically a pre-60s discourse that hasn't even caught up with Black Power or Goffman and the sociology of deviance, not to mention postmodernism generally, postcolonial studies, subaltern studies, queer theory, critical race theory, etc. You can easily argue that GA is a cult in a capsule. If we don't do some catching up soon, as Suryia points out, we're not going to have any sort of claim to be considered as a serious psychosocial discourse.

You can go back to James Anthony and Pat de Maré for the importance of structure. The structure of GA trainings remains a problem, not least in the way that those in charge cling to it and the way it shapes marginalisation. Authoritarian structures facilitate authoritarian processes and keep everyone stuck, including those of us stuck on the margins.

Bw,
Dick

From: Claire Bacha
Date: 14 October 2021, 7:23
To: Dick Blackwell

Dear Dick,

Hannah Arendt says that once an action has been taken, it cannot be taken back. We lose control of it. This is akin to Elias' (1991) ideas about figurations of ideas and actions of individuals and groups in relation to each other evolving through time. These are profound ideas at the heart of group-analytic theory and practice. It does not matter that the people who wrote about this are dead. They are important ideas in decolonizing from neoliberalism. I am grateful to Farhad for drawing my attention to Elias. Elias was an important part of the beginning of group analysis and part of our ongoing group analytic ideas, including how we might use other ideas, like intersectionality, in our work. Our psychosocial discourse is different from others because of this.

Indeed, because of Arendt, Elias and Foulkes, and other knowledge, I no longer think in terms of structures. Understanding processes is more important. Change is ubiquitous. If something is not changing, there is something else keeping it from changing or keeping it in balance. That is not to say that we like change. Humans also need homeostasis (rather than stasis). Stasis is not healthy, as we know therapeutically. Arendt, Elias and Foulkes point to a different way of thinking about things. It is a different motivator of action, perhaps a more peaceful one if it saves lives and energy but allows change.

The other, more structural, works that you mention are important, too. My critique here is that they do not recognize the importance of groups and how groups foster potential for personal and interpersonal integration. Clinical work teaches us this, and we largely keep it to ourselves. I agree that we need more of a dialogue with these other ways of thinking. Maybe Foulkes, Arendt and Elias need to be taught together at the university level, or earlier.

My main preoccupation in the IGA, though, is how to have an organization that uses group-analytic concepts creatively. This is more difficult than one would have thought. The IGA is not immune to pressures from the outside world. If we work to resolve the problems in the IGA, this will help us understand more about the world that we are living in and being creative in that world.

I am chair of the PPP group on student experience. I would love to hear your ideas on how to improve it. What are your ideas about areas of stasis in the IGA?

Bw,
Claire

From: Dick Blackwell
Date: 26 October 2021, 19:50
To: Claire Bacha

Dear Claire,

Re: Arendt: I think the Macbeths had a similar experience of action that cannot be taken back, leading to loss of control. But I can't see what either Arendt or Elias contributes to ideas of decolonisation. 'The Established and the Outsiders' (Elias and Scotston, 1965); its 'gossip' is essentially about conscious prejudice. Decolonisation has to be addressed to structures and social-unconscious processes.

I can't see how our GA psychosocial discourse is different from other psychosocial discourses. I think you're heading for a frequent safe haven for GAs: keeping the discussion abstract, protected from contact with the real world. Talking about 'change' and 'homeostasis' and abstract distinctions between 'process' and 'structure' without applying them to concrete issues serve that purpose. For example, I can't see how one addresses food banks without considering the structure of the benefits system and the part it plays in the wider structure of class exploitation, which includes anti-TU legislation. Process is essentially constrained by structure. I also don't understand how postmodernism, cultural studies, post-colonial studies, etc., are to be viewed as relating to structure, not process. They arose from the exhaustion of the old-left's base-superstructure paradigm.

Re: the student experience group. At present, I issue health warnings to all potential students who are Black or working class – or those who are both and thereby in twice as much danger. My 2018 article spells out how the 'Welcome to our club – as long as you become like us and don't make an issue of your difference' works (Blackwell, 2018). It was elaborated by Guilaine (Kinouani, 2020a, 2020b) in Stuart's recent article on positionality (Stevenson, 2020) and by Anne (Aiyegbusi, 2021a, 2021b), Suryia (Nayak, 2021a, 2021b) and Jacinta (Kent, 2021) wrote.

The student experience would be improved if all staff were familiar with this. 'Teaching' staff apparently don't read the journal. Moreover, they need some idea about how being white shapes their view of the world. Staff should reflect on how little we find on reading lists of what has been written in the journal on race and culture in the last 30 years and how much responsibility they're prepared to take for it. But, most important, as I keep saying and you keep missing, would be to give them power. That's real power over what they learn and how they learn it – and how they're assessed. It remains very hierarchical and authoritarian, not at all GA. The main complaint I've heard from both black and white students is that they're infantilised and their prior knowledge, experience and expertise disrespected. That, from an educational point of view, suggests a reactionary model. I suggest that all your committee and all 'teaching staff' in any GA institute read Freire's *Pedagogy of the Oppressed* (1996) to find the possibilities of genuinely mutual educational relationships between staff and students.

Reading your response to Farhad (Bacha, 2021), you seem unfamiliar with alternative models of supervision and assessment, most notably the one pioneered by Meg Sharpe and written up in the journal in the 1980s (Sharpe and Blackwell, 1987).

Bw,
Dick

From: Claire Bacha
Date: 30 October 2021, 9:47
To: Dick Blackwell

Dear Dick,

What do Arendt and Elias contribute to decolonization in terms of ideas? First, let me say that I enjoyed Guilaine's (Kinouani, 2020a, 2020b) papers immensely. Her ideas about decolonization in group analysis chime with other ideas about how we decolonize from neoliberalism. Arendt and Elias do not focus on decolonization. However, they show how we might think outside of colonialism and neoliberalism. This is the possibility of another world being born. They are different from most other psychosocial discourses in two ways. One, they are dialectical, like Foulkes. Two, they are about the working of groups (not just a vague 'social' v. 'individual'). They combine well with Foulkes, giving a space for group-analytic concepts to be relevant and applicable to life outside the consulting room. The Established and the Outsiders, for example, put us in contact with ideas about elements that stop the integration of newness and difference in communities, thus allowing us to be more conscious about these processes and how to counter them. I think that The Established and the Outsiders, and gossip, are relevant to what stops change. If you are calling the change 'decolonization', then it is directly relevant to what you want to achieve. I don't think that these processes are all conscious.

Yes, you are right about structure and process being like figure and ground. The reason I choose to think more in terms of process is the enhanced thought processes that go with assuming that things change and then looking for what stops them from changing and in whose interests. It makes me feel more powerful about making the changes that need to be made. It directs my thoughts in more specific, practical ways. It seems to me that you are addressing food banks in a process way. We need both structure and process as humans. At this moment, clearly, there are structures stopping global changes we need, as with the environment.

We can also ask: what changes do we need to make in the IGA? What stops them from happening? What structures do we need in order to do what we need to do? How do they conflict with each other, and where can they be discussed? What needs changed, and what needs preserved?

This brings me to the student experience group. I am interested that you lobby against it with the very people who might be interested in it and those who might need it. I am interested in it because I am interested in the experiences of students. Is it me that you are objecting to when you lobby against it? To be more specific, you are assuming that I am involved in 'authoritarian teaching'. I don't think that you have ever looked into what happens in Manchester. Teaching there is student-led. Students present; the staff member is there to facilitate. I always learned just as much or more than the students. It is a great way to teach and learn.

Talking about the power of students and change, the group was instrumental in creating the national students' group. It looks at other ways of integrating minorities, hearing their training experiences, putting them in touch with each other and helping them to speak truth to power. Other PPP initiatives include decolonizing the curriculum and whiteness groups. We are working on a revised Workbook in Group Analysis based on intersectionality. Our issue of the journal on racism promotes these ideas.

In the group, I listen to the experiences of our students of colour and colleagues and learn from them. I have invited you to share your ideas with us. If all you can do is lobby against the group because of your own blind spots and prejudices, I have to see this as more destructive than constructive. I don't want to see you this way because I have a lot of respect for you. You have a right to say, 'I told you so'. But it is not right of you to destroy the very things that you have been working for and with. I would like to hear your objections to the group. Do you really think that I am stopping things from happening?

I do, though, support the uses of authority in supervision and, especially, in therapy. Maybe this is where a further dialogue needs to take place. I see therapy as the central element of our training. Many people come to training for the therapy, and it is our responsibility to preserve the therapeutic space and make it safe. I think that the supervision space is similar. Hearing that these spaces have not been safe for our students of colour is serious and must be listened to. This is why I am in the group. There should be more staff members in it – and students, too.

The role of authority in therapy and supervision is crucial to the quality of the therapy the students receive and the therapy that they can give. This is where I differ from you and Farhad. If we do not have authority, we cannot use it to look at the transferences and countertransferences that make up the therapy, as well as the interactions between equals. We use a particular kind of leadership in our therapy groups, and we teach it. We are hoping to model good-enough authority. Power does not have to be misused. A lot of what goes on in therapy and supervision is about the possibility of receiving and providing a good-enough power that facilitates people becoming themselves with others: their internal and social integration. I may not be putting this well, but this is how therapy worked for me.

Best regards,
Claire

From: Dick Blackwell
Date: 2 November 2021, 19:29
To: Claire Bacha

Claire, I'm not aware I'm lobbying against the student experience group. I may be challenging it by asking, 'are you serious about change?' But I don't understand what 'lobbying against it' means.

We certainly disagree about power. In my view, Acton was right when he said, 'all power corrupts'. Two thousand years of history, and all before it, supports that claim. The only thing that legitimates power is its accountability to those over whom it is exercised. That's the basis of historical ideas about 'democracy', the basis of most organisational constitutions where members elect the governing body. I understand it as the cornerstone of Arendt's philosophy. Machiavelli, too, saw political justice and stability as dependent on a balance of power between competing interest groups. I don't believe all the competing interests in the world or in UK 'society' are reconcilable.

You talked about being colonised by neoliberalism. But neoliberalism depends on the unopposed power of the managers of capital and their media allies. That's behind the draconian legislation against Trade Unions that has existed for nearly 40 years. The market must be 'free' except for one thing: no freedom for workers to organise and bargain collectively over pay, conditions and the running of the organisation.

You talk about the training in Manchester being student-led since students present, but I'm asking about who determines what gets presented and, most importantly, what part students play in assessment. Because if the decision about who qualifies is in the hands of the staff, then that power relationship shapes all interactions. What suggests the group looks at what Meg Sharpe and I wrote (Sharpe and Blackwell, 1987) and thinks about whether there is a problem with that sort of empowerment of students? Who benefits from the deskilling?

I don't think you need power and authority for transference and countertransference. They're ubiquitous. But I do think the need for power and authority is what leads to GA and other forms of therapy to become technologies of social control rather than a praxis of liberation. It's also what enabled the persistence (for about 40 years and still counting) of the practice of analysts interpreting analysands' accounts of their experiences of racism as displacements of something else.

I'm not looking to integrate newness. I'm looking to expand and diversify a culture and take multiculturalism more seriously. GA is still monocultural. Decolonising is about expanding minds constrained by colonial thinking derived from colonial processes and structures, especially authority structures. Have a look at Okeke's (Azu-Okeke, 2003) response to my lecture, and you can see what I mean. I don't think in terms of 'decolonial ideas' so much as decolonising as a praxis of deconstructing colonial culture and colonial mindsets as they are manifested in Western psychotherapy. Since colonialism and capitalism are so interwoven and so much part of each other, I think deconstructing capitalism is more meaningful than simply being anticapitalist. I'm not convinced capitalism has to be abolished, but it does have to be severely constrained. When does a restaurant or a chain of half a dozen start to develop into McDonalds?

Bw,
Dick

From: Claire Bacha
Date: 3 November 2021, 7:44
To: Dick Blackwell

Dear Dick,

Lobbying is an American term that formalizes the expression of sectional interests in the 'lobby' of the American Congress.
On 26 Oct 2021, at 19:50, Dick Blackwell wrote:

'Re: the student experience group. At present, I issue health warnings to all potential students who are Black or working class or – those who are both who are thereby in twice as much danger.'

This looks like lobbying to me. You are lobbying against PPP by 'issuing a health warning to . . . those who are . . . in danger'. This is a different question from 'Are you serious about change?'

Am I serious about change? Well, yes, some changes. I love group analysis as a theory and practice, and I don't want to throw the baby out with the bathwater. What I am serious about is making sure students get the best experience possible, attracting and retaining a diverse student body that feels able to contribute from themselves, preventing abuses of power, position and privilege.

I am also serious about using what group analysis has taught us to create a group-analytic organization in the IGA, and particularly to create a group analysis that can become a new model of democratic processes and organization, which is badly needed. I think that this is the realization of the work that began with Foulkes and Elias. There are other modalities and other forms of action. We have a specific technique and theory that has an important place among them, capable of helping to create and maintain a new world. I don't want the kernel of group analysis to be overwhelmed with these other modalities. Students come to us because they are attracted by group analysis as a modality of thinking and action, as well as therapy. We need to preserve that kernel.

This kernel is a specific form of work with power and authority. We do a good job with authority, I think. Part of our training is to teach us how to always step down from bringing our own concerns into the group, except when the group needs to hear them. We also train to step down from the idealization and omnipotence that can be attributed to us. Sometimes, we need to hold it, but without believing it ourselves. This is difficult. We teach self-care as an important part of doing the superhuman job of containing feelings and enabling connections between thoughts and feelings. We train to make use of supervision as a vital component of being able to do this superhuman job socially, with the help of others. It is a difficult job, and often, we are dealing with our own reactions to powerlessness. We need authority not to produce transference and countertransference, which, as you say, happens anyway, but to avoid pushing the authority issues away, to contain them and not act on them. We won't get rid of authority. It is in our evolutionary histories and in our current forms of family and childcare. We can only learn how to deal with it to create a belief in good authority in ourselves and in our trainees and patients. Not all authority is good. We also need to learn to recognize authority that is being misused and to speak truth to power, which means holding our own authority.

I also think that we are becoming better at power exactly because we are listening to our students and acting. I am speaking for PPP as a whole here. Acton did not say, 'All power corrupts'. Acton (1887) said something much more complex and accurate: 'Power tends to corrupt and absolute power corrupts absolutely'. We need to do more work on power as an emotional process that starts with the powerlessness of the baby. We also need to find ways of having a better democracy that counters the corrupting process of power. I am glad that you explained your process a bit more to me. I don't think that group analysis and psychoanalysis are colonial ideas in their entirety. They are, at their base, a creation of a reaction to antisemitism. You should read my paper with Sue Einhorn on antisemitism (Bacha et al., 2021). There are some insights about humans that just *are*. These can be used in different ways. We are talking about powerful ideas that are highly countercultural and can illuminate processes and help us to construct something new. That is beyond deconstruction. I think we need both. Deconstruction does not happen without ideas about what might arise from it. What kind of world do we want? At our best, we empower people to be able to speak to each other about the worlds that they want and why. People able to think and act together is the best kind of power. I just want us to be at our best.

In fact, I think that the journal issue on Racism shows us at our best. It is just a first step.

Bw,
Claire

References

Acton (1887) Letter to Archbishop Mandell Creighton.

Aiyegbusi, A. (2021a) The White Mirror: Face to Face with Racism in Group Analysis Part 1 – Mainly Theory. *Group Analysis*, 54(3): 402–420. https://doi.org/10.1177/0533316421992315

Aiyegbusi, A. (2021b) The White Mirror: Face to Face with Racism in Group Analysis Part 2 – Mainly Practice. *Group Analysis*, 54(3): 421–436. https://doi.org/10.1177/0533316421992438

Andrews, K. (2018) *Back to Black: Retelling Black Radicalism for the 21st Century*. London: Zed Books.

Arendt, H. (1951) *The Origins of Totalitarianism*. New York: Harcourt, Brace and Cia.

Arendt, H. (1998) *The Human Condition*. Chicago: University of Chicago Press.

Azu-Okeke, O. (2003) Response to Lecture by Dick Blackwell. *Group Analysis*, 36(4): 465–476. https://doi.org/10.1177/0533316403364003

Bacha, C. S. (2021) Response to Farad Dalal's 'The Ethics of Supervision'. *Group Analysis*: 053331642110507. https://doi.org/10.1177/05333164211050779

Bacha, C. S., Einhorn, S. and Lieberman, S. (2021) 'If You Prick Me, Do I Not Bleed?': Antisemitism, Racism and Group Analysis – Some Thoughts. *Group Analysis*, 54(3): 388–401. https://doi.org/10.1177/0533316421996111

Blackwell, D. (1988) Group Analysis, Mediation and Transcontextuality. *Group Analysis*, 21(2): 181–188. https://doi.org/10.1177/0533316488212012

Blackwell, D. (1994) The Emergence of Racism in Group Analysis. *Group Analysis*, 27(2): 197–210. https://doi.org/10.1177/0533316494272006

Blackwell, D. (2003) Colonialism and Globalization: A Group-Analytic Perspective. *Group Analysis*, 36(4): 445–463. https://doi.org/10.1177/0533316403364002

Blackwell, D. (2018) Cultural Transition, Negation and the Social Unconscious. *Group Analysis*, 51(3): 304–314. https://doi.org/10.1177/0533316418791102

Blackwell, D. (2020) The Impenetrable Wall of Whiteness. A Response to Guilaine Kinouani. *Group Analysis*, 53(1): 92–101. https://doi.org/10.1177/0533316419890176

Borossa, J. (2021) Special Issue: Racism. *Group Analysis*, 54(3).

Burman, E. (2021) Frantz Fanon and Revolutionary Group Praxis. *Group Analysis*, 54(2): 169–188. https://doi.org/10.1177/05333164211001192

Dalal, F. N. (1993) 'Race' and Racism: An Attempt to Organize Difference. *Group Analysis*, 26(3): 277–290. https://doi.org/10.1177/0533316493263008

Dalal, F. N. (2015) Group Analytic Training and the Social Context: Who Is Influencing Whom? *Group Analysis*, 48(3): 349–367. https://doi.org/10.1177/0533316415600624

Dalal, F. N. (2021) The Ethics of Supervision: Reciprocity, Emergence and Prefiguration. *Group Analysis*: 053331642110507. https://doi.org/10.1177/05333164211050756

Elias, N. (1991) *The Society of Individuals*. New York: Continuum.

Elias, N. and Scotston, J. (1965) *The Established and the Outsiders: A Sociological Enquiry into Community Problems*. London: F Cass.

Freire, P. (1996) *Pedagogy of the Oppressed*. London: Penguin Books.

Hopper, E. (2018) The Development of the Concept of the Tripartite Matrix: A Response to 'Four Modalities of the Experience of Others in Groups' by Victor Schermer. *Group Analysis*, 51(2): 197–206.

Illich, I. (1971) *Deschooling Society*. London: Calder & Boyars.

Kent, J. (2021) Scapegoating and the 'Angry Black Woman'. *Group Analysis*, 54(3): 354–371. https://doi.org/10.1177/0533316421992300

Kinouani, G. (2020a) Difference, Whiteness and the Group Analytic Matrix: An Integrated Formulation. *Group Analysis*, 53(1): 60–74. https://doi.org/10.1177/0533316419883455

Kinouani, G. (2020b) Silencing, Power and Racial Trauma in Groups. *Group Analysis*, 53(2): 145–161. https://doi.org/10.1177/0533316420908974

Morton, A. (1989) *A People's History of England*. London: Lawrence & Wishart.

Nayak, S. (2021a) Black Feminist Intersectionality Is Vital to Group Analysis: Can Group Analysis Allow Outsider Ideas In? *Group Analysis*, 54(3): 337–353. https://doi.org/10.1177/0533316421997767

Nayak, S. (2021b) Racialized Misogyny: Response to 44th Foulkes Lecture. *Group Analysis*, 54(4): 520–527. https://doi.org/10.1177/05333164211039983

Novak, T. (1988) *Poverty and the State*. Milton Keynes: Open University Press.

Sharpe, M. and Blackwell, D. (1987) Creative Supervision through Student Involvement. *Group Analysis*, 20(3): 195–208. https://doi.org/10.1177/0533316487203001

Stevenson, S. (2020) Psychodynamic Intersectionality and the Positionality of the Group Analyst: The Tension Between Analytical Neutrality and Inter-Subjectivity. *Group Analysis*, 53(4): 498–514. https://doi.org/10.1177/0533316420953660

Conclusion

A Group-Analytic Intersectional Manifesto

Alasdair Forrest

There is a disquiet alive in Group Analysis: a recognition that power, privilege, and position have been under-examined in terms of their operation in the lives of patients, students, and group therapists. How Group Analysis develops now will significantly influence group therapy more broadly, particularly psychodynamic group therapy. At the centre of any change, though, stands the Foulkesian idea that individuals are social to their core. Therapeutic groups, too, are ineluctably bound up in these social forces, which continuously reproduce themselves:

> *Psychotherapy groups are not isolated rafts floating adrift in a vacuum. . . . Groups are full of people with lives in the world . . . and the group analyst refers constantly in his or her mind to his/her own dominant theoretical discourse.*

> (Dalal, 1998:177)

As the Institute of Group Analysis is mobilised by this, in particular through the Power, Position, and Privilege Group (PPP), there is a possibility of change. This requires a turning towards strong feelings, rather than a turning away, recognising as Shelhi does in this volume: 'the anger of the oppressed "is loaded with information and energy" (Lorde, 2019:121).

The central problem of how to mobilise these concepts, addressed in this volume, comes in three questions, stated by Nayak in the introduction, and which can now be restated, with more emphasis, as a challenge:

- How does intersectionality enable anti-racist therapeutic group work?
- How are theoretical exchanges between intersectionality and Group Analysis contributing to explorations of inevitable issues of power, position, and privilege in group-analytic training, practice, and organisation – and in what ways is that not happening? How can we change it if not?
- Doesn't the relationship between intersectionality and Group Analysis demonstrate the necessity for Group Analysis to allow its slow, open theoretical group to accommodate outsider concepts?

DOI: 10.4324/9781003232216-9

There is, nonetheless, a risk of lip service and tokenism, adding intersectional words to group-analytic concepts, or even, as Blackwell states in this volume, "putting Kimberlé Crenshaw, bell hooks and Angela Davis, and indeed Suryia Nayak and Anne Aiyegbusi, on a reading list" while changing little else. This would impoverish the field while also failing to provide a space that allows this essential conceptualisation of how human lives are constrained and traumatised by the operation of axes of power, thus failing patients who dwell in these intersections.

In parallel to Spivak's (1988) caution, it would leave the field trying to inaugurate a Black queer feminist perspective in Group Analysis, for example, yet just reproducing the same exclusion and marginalisation with a different set of words.

In probably the classic work of post-colonial theory, which has a broader relevance to many forms of thinking, Spivak writes of a concealed Western subject that is always at play in discourses on, in, and of India in particular, or the post-colonial world in general. She argues that an attempt to somehow provide a voice for the working-class women of post-colonial countries she describes is merely a cover for continually maintaining Western authority over the discourse. However, simply listening to voices from people who are constituted at a pole of being oppressed in one or more ways does not resolve the problem if there is not a whole-group confrontation with the processes of exclusion and oppression in which all take part – including unwittingly. The clinical, training, and theory-making processes in group analysis need to find a way to be hospitable to these outsider ideas not merely by finding a place for them – certainly not in a module on Critical Group Analysis – but instead need to be grappled with continuously as the field develops (Forrest and Nayak, 2021).

As Benjamin says, quoting Lorde, the master's tools will never demolish the master's house – and new, intersectional tools are needed. If not, the words may change, but the syntax, language – and syntactical foreclosures about what cannot possibly be meant or made sense of – would remain the same.

Benjamin says that the group reflects the conductor's own fragmented identities. There is work to be done. In the same way, Group Analysis may well reflect the fragmented identities of its theory-makers and theory-reproducers. Again, there is work to be done. This needs to be different if a different way of listening and responding is possible. This work is unsettling and involves a substantial re-examination: "An anti-racist or black feminist group analysis is not white group analysis in blackface" (Nayak, 2021). Indeed, something that liberates people to express their experience cannot have the same constraining structure that operates throughout people's lives. It is, therefore, clear that a clinically-focused account, although it gains from its clinical roots, but one that involves a change in word choice alone, will do little to allow the possibility of therapeutic change.

Conversely, the discipline could lose itself in theorising without clinical work being at the centre of that theory, failing to use it to explain anything. Empty theory is not needed. Psychotherapy is not a discursive discipline on the page. It is an affectively-engaged discipline about change. In this volume, this comes alive as Shelhi writes in her discussion of affectivism, or as Aiyegbusi demonstrates so vividly with the clinical work with female offender-patients and with the discussions in supervision. It comes alive in the bodily focus in the accounts of the clinical work of Anderson and Benjamin. It involves people who are suffering and seeking some exploration of their difficulties with the hope of better lives.

Instead of indulging in any kind of wordplay, in this volume, authors have articulated a perspective on human distress that recognises and engages creatively with the group-analytic literature and with the literature in queer theory, Black feminism, feminist science studies – and, in sum, intersectionality – while grounding what is considered in the clinical experience of group therapy, as patient and as conductor, or as both.

Authors have addressed themselves to:

1 Clinical practice
2 Group-analytic training
3 Developing a methodology for theorising that is more intersectional

They have done so with the kinds of intersectional questions Nayak posed in the introduction in mind. As a conclusion, I shall review these areas with reference to those crucial questions for our discipline at this time. In doing so, though, it becomes clear that any account is incomplete. If we are suggesting that people are constituted by multiple axes of power relationships, it surely becomes impossible to be complete in the account given. This is familiar to Group Analysts, where it rarely feels like a complete truth appears in the group. Instead, there is a continuous, increasingly complex unfolding.

The authors, for example, continue implicitly to address the issue of class as another axis of intersectional identity – but rarely do so explicitly. That may be in part because, in the United Kingdom, class is so interwoven into our view of our national life that it remains implicit in all our interactions: a social unconscious phenomenon that is a set of "arrangements [that] are not perceived (not 'known'), and if perceived, not acknowledged ('denied'), and if acknowledged, not taken as problematic ('given'), and if taken as problematic, not considered with an optimal degree of detachment and objectivity" (Hopper, 1996).

I. Clinical Practice

How does intersectionality enable anti-racist therapeutic group work?

Intersectionality, by its nature, involves a holding together of things that could be fragmented. This is in the individual, and in the group, and in their interaction.

Aiyegbusi says that intersectionality can provide "a particular anti-discriminatory rigour" to group-analytic work. She argues for a reconceptualisation of the group matrix as an intersectional matrix containing "immediate and ancestral nationality, age, religion, race, culture, ethnicity, gender and sexual identity, class, physical health and ability, family structures, educational and professional achieve-ments, personal and generational, structural and interpersonal traumatogenic and criminogenic factors". This provides a basis for considering the dynamic matrix as it evolves in terms of enactments borne of those intersectional positions. For example, she describes criminal, even offence-paralleling interactions as being possible but as being best understood (most of all by the individual responsible) in the intersectional context. She argues that this robustly holds together aspects of the individual identity that can be fragmented and, in that way, holds promise for a kind of justice, or at least a hearing, that does more than recapitulate problems.

In a different context, Anderson argues that the holding together must not only be for each person but also for the group-as-a-whole. Arguing for group polyphony, he says that a group best attends to equality of voices, where there is no one truth, and where silencing (and marginalisation or pathologisation) is to be resisted relentlessly.

Benjamin joins this call, saying that the "weathered bodies" of members of oppressed groups become so largely through projective identification. Just as I write that the process of working on this requires a recognition of the whole group's disa-vowals, she mentions this albeit more explicitly. She argues strongly for a centring of the mind-body connection and an open recognition of the intersection of trauma, poverty, power(lessness), privilege, and historical oppression. Her description of the historical process of the oppression of Black women, in particular, chimes with Anderson's description of psychotherapists' pathologisation of gay people and with Dizadji's description of the processes of her own forced political exile.

For all of the authors, the start of a solution comes, then, in recognising that context produces identities. It comes in holding these different identities in a person and held together in the group – but most of all, being made explicit rather than disavowed.

In an attempt to be very explicit, Nayak (2022) proposes four tasks to prompt intersectional thinking and hold in mind conscious and unconscious intersectional dynamics:

- Name the roads of social inequality and how they crisscross.
- Name the vehicles of oppression on roads of social inequality.
- Describe the crash/collision at the intersection.
- Describe the bio-psycho-social injuries.

This programme is restated here to provide an outline to guide those looking to start to orientate themselves to intersectional aspects of what happens in groups. It is grounded in a metaphor related to traffic that comes from the work of Crenshaw (1989). It helps the group analyst to consider intersecting axes of oppression and consider how they are driven while also considering in an embodied and relational way the outcome of these intersections.

How are theoretical exchanges with intersectionality developing group-analytic practice? Doesn't this show the need for openness to outsider concepts?

Theoretical exchanges between intersectionality and group-analytic practice come alive in the work of the authors. All maintain an explicitly Foulkesian basis for their work – some with more sense of ambivalence than others. The encounter with intersectionality has caused them to re-examine the concepts of mirroring and resonance, the matrix, and the nature of exchange in groups.

Benjamin argues that empathic attunement to an individual's experience is impossible if their intersectional experiences of being othered are not attuned to. She suggests that containment is not possible without this being open to being contained in the mind of the conductor. Similarly, but with a focus more on power in society rather than Benjamin's explicit rooting of her theory in bodies, Dizadji and Nayak articulate clearly the need for intersectional aspects of traumatisation to be considered fully in the context of the political operation of oppressive power, if therapeutic work is to be possible in those who have survived extreme traumatisation. They call therapy political by its nature since human relations are political and intersectional by their nature.

This is the thickest segment of a thread that runs through the book, where complex statements of identity can be made and held together and referred to historical trends and current political choices. These are affectively-laden aspects of identity and oppression, though, and as a result, affect is never far from the concepts the authors find helpful.

Perhaps predictably, given the observation that difference can be the site of disturbance in the group, several authors problematise the idea of location of disturbance. Foulkes used the term in two ways: both as the place where disturbance originated at that time, even if that was not manifest initially, and as the process of making a location of disturbance, so the group analyst interpreting this, possibly iteratively. Anderson divides these two meanings somewhat as part of a commitment to avoid pathologising that comes, in part, from recognising the way that gay people have been pathologised in psychoanalytic circles and their difference treated as a disturbance.

Anderson writes that

> a group analyst . . . must take seriously [his] caution regarding the location of difference not becoming the location of disturbance. A group must democratically and equally deconstruct such meanings, thereby pushing each member of the group, and the group analyst, into new and sometimes uncomfortable speaking positions as it finds and problematises locations of difference and similarity.

With a different emphasis, Shelhi sees affectivism as a way of responding to feelings about intersectional experiences of oppression. She combines a sense of affect with one of activism to form the idea. It involves turning towards rather than away from difficult emotion, and similarly to Anderson involves taking a "curious rather than curative approach" [her emphasis] towards locations of disturbance, seeing them as potential locations of discovery.

In an echo of my comments on Spivak, she shows from painful experience that simply speaking is not the matter at hand. Shelhi found little difficulty in word choice or even in using her voice. She writes articulately about her experience and how it came to be what it was. The difficulty came in the affective figuration that surrounded it and in a feeling of lack of solidarity and lack of awareness of oppressive ways of relating.

Shelhi proposes attention to *"felt-sense split-second moments* of someone's dignity being compromised or integrity violated" and says that "naming something is in itself an intervention". If group-analytic practice is starting to see that identities are intersectional, that in itself is not enough. Group analysts need ways of attending to these experiences in ways that are like those suggested by Anderson and Shelhi.

Nayak and Dizadji's mention of locational intersectionality, and Aiyegbusi's restatement of the matrix as an intersectional matrix, described in what follows, have as much relevance to clinical practice as they do to theoretical development. That is the nature of a field where theory and practice can never be distinct.

Indeed, in my chapter, I describe how my practice has changed as my thinking around diffraction has developed, such that I take a stance as a conductor that is more active around helping recognise points of alignment. I am not certain that this is right, but it is where my practice currently is. I argue that the potential for marginalisation and silencing around marginalised intersectional identities is so great that it cannot be left to the trust of the group alone and requires the work of the conductor. This is similar in nature, albeit of course not in degree, to how Dizadji and Nayak describe the work with torture survivors, where the stance of the conductor to extreme traumatisation is necessarily different. I think this is because of the way traumatisation separates people from any sense of a human collective membership.

2.   Group Analytic Training

How does intersectionality enable anti-racist therapeutic group-analytic training?

The authors who address training as a major part of their contribution are clear in their views that training has some way to go to be anti-racist. Indeed, some authors have questioned the extent to which the attempts to de-centre Whiteness and provide a safe training space for Black students are possible with the current structures and attitudes. Blackwell, in particular, argues from this position – while his correspondent, Bacha, holds more optimism for the possibility of dialogue and change, saying that her priority is to have the organisations use group-analytic concepts creatively.

Blackwell puts his priorities starkly:

In the wider world of psychoanalysis and psychoanalytic psychotherapy, some of us have spent decades challenging a status quo in which black analysands routinely have their experiences of racism denied and reassigned to something else by their analysts. Most Black psychotherapy students have a painful and

*alienating experience. . . . I expect the Black women pioneers I'm not in touch
with suffer something similar. Black students coming to train these days need to
be given a health warning: 'This training can do you damage!'*

Bacha argues against throwing out the baby with the bathwater of what group analysis and training in it are not currently doing. She says that she has seen the IGA
move from "a more participatory and chaotic organization" to something more
managerial, but says that she can see a way forward towards improving participation. She says that decolonising the curriculum in group-analytic training is possible, and an effort is underway. Blackwell replies that he thinks decolonising the
curriculum alone is not enough. He says that the institutional power, represented,
for example, in the panel of readers who approve or refer back qualifying papers,
is the site of significant resistance to change.

The PPP group came about from students' descriptions of difficulties in confront-
ing these issues, and from early on, it has had current students involved heavily in
its work. Shelhi describes some of the difficulties needing to be addressed, too, in
a highly personal account infused with the bodily feeling that is characteristic of
intersectional writers. She described the disavowal of connection and solidarity:

*Situations where I became the location of disturbance for expressing opinions that
weren't sanctioned by the mainstream. When, behind the scenes, people expressed
quiet solidarity, I often wanted to say, "Why didn't you speak up then?".*

There is a risk that people will simply "make agreeable noises to get through [their]
training", as she says. Instead, the unfinished position put forward by the authors
is something more akin to refusing to ignore oppressive dynamics and finding a
way to be certain that they are likely and are not absent simply by their seeming
absence, which may be instead about a disavowal. This is not resolved – and there
is a sense that this is always likely to be a process of conflictual moving towards a
resolution – but it is in the theoretical exchange that progress could emerge.

*How are theoretical exchanges with intersectionality developing group-analytic
training? Doesn't this show the need for openness to outsider concepts?*

Inasmuch as students could make agreeable noises to get through their training, the
training could make agreeable noises to get through their students. The majority
of Bacha and Blackwell's exchange focuses on an unresolved pair of positions. As
noted previously, Blackwell is highly sceptical that there can be a meaningful change
without a major change in personal relations at the political level as well as major
organisational change. His programme is revolutionary. Bacha's is different: saying
that things can be done and be meaningful, that theory can change, and that group
analysts are "experts in group conversations" who can put this expertise to use.

Bacha refers to changes in the IGA curriculum being proposed through the
Power, Position, and Privilege group and extends an invitation to join in her

exchange with Blackwell. As experienced staff members in the training, they turn to the constraints on the training imposed from all its contexts. They do not seem to be addressing the question of whether these concepts are relevant. That is taken as accepted. Here, they are closest in their position.

Their contributions resonate with those of Aiyegbusi and Benjamin, who both refer to the historical injustices that are alive in relationships in the group matrix or in the body – but focus explicitly on the training. Both refer to historical processes and the current operation of political power in the context of the IGA, referring to capitalism and neoliberalism and their permeation of the organisation.

Indeed, Bacha argues that "all our minds are colonised by neoliberalism". She has written before about the way that group-analytic organisations struggle to remain group-analytic in their character in the context of new public management and the regulatory environment (Bacha, 2015). Blackwell, though, bemoans the theoretical position of Group Analysis, which he describes as "pre-60s".

Perhaps inevitably, eventually, the discussion is about power. It is here that there is the most unresolved aspect of the group-analytic training. Blackwell argues that

> the need for power and authority is what leads to GA and other forms of therapy to become technologies of social control rather than a praxis of liberation. It's also what enabled the persistence (for about 40 years and still counting) of the practice of analysts interpreting analysands' accounts of their experiences of racism as displacements of something else.

Bacha argues instead that, through the PPP group and other things, group analysts are "becoming better at power". She suggests that changes do come a step at a time and that the important thing is to give students a good experience in a situation where the Institute has democratic characteristics so that power is used properly.

This all chimes, again, with Spivak's observations. There is no disagreement among the authors as to whether intersectional concepts are helpful. The disagreement seems to be whether they can come into the training and remain intersectional concepts since they must not remain just as concepts but instead must infuse an entire approach that includes not just the curriculum but recruitment of staff, selection of students, and marking of qualifying papers.

3.   Developing a Model of Theorising That Is More Intersectional

How does intersectionality enable anti-racist theoretical development in group therapy? How are theoretical exchanges with intersectionality developing group-analytic theory-making? Doesn't this show the need for openness to outsider concepts?

In my chapter, I cite the review of the work of Donna Haraway, with its further development in that review by Campbell (2004). Haraway talks about diffraction rather than reflection. I argue that groups work best when the conductor can think with and develop a diffractive perspective, with various points of connection and difference held in mind. I further argue that the mirror reaction is a two-dimensional idea that does not suit conditions of intersectional exclusion and oppression. In a paper focused on the therapeutic group, I do not talk explicitly about a model for developing a new theory. However, I do show where applying or failing to apply this model has been helpful or unhelpful. This work of the individual conductor is a start.

There is a more developed example of this happening in action in supervision between the two clinicians in Aiyegbusi's chapter, where they must recognise the intersectional differences between each other in order to effectively work with the group as co-therapists. This kind of in-the-moment theorising, linked to specific clinical experience, is the groundwork for theory production on the page and in the seminar. Aiyegbusi shows us that analytic theory cannot be developed in a top-down way alone but rather in a bottom-up way. In this regard, group analysts have much to offer Intersectional writers who do not have day-to-day contact with therapeutic group work, with all its potential, albeit imperfect, for attending to relational dynamics.

In preparing this book, the authors met several times online. They shared experiences about the problems and opportunities of writing, as well as sharing ideas they were considering writing about or developing. They considered the intersectional difficulties in finding one's voice. They noticed resonances between the theoretical ideas being described and developed. This kind of discussion is key to developing a theory that is not about borders (my idea, your idea) but instead about a shared grappling towards something. In the introduction, Nayak cites the Combahee River Collective. She, I, and other authors also cite Crenshaw's work, which involved organising of marginalised groups into legal class actions. In the history of Black feminism, which is the origin of Intersectionality, ideas have often come from collaboration and collective action – in short, from discussion, including very personal, affective discussion – and not solely from an individual articulation.

The small groups contained possible authors who were not able to continue with the project, and their contributions were valuable in helping the authors who were able to contribute in thinking about their work. Equally, some authors joined later, like in a slow-open group, and their different experiences of the conversations illuminated thinking.

This kind of work is exemplified in the written dialogue between Nayak and Dizadji, which developed from the group, and in the edited internet dialogue between Blackwell and Bacha. Nayak and Dizadji are able to illuminate each other's contributions and build on them, almost walking together through a path towards thinking about traumatisation. Blackwell and Bacha do not come to an agreement – and indeed disagree on whether they are having a dialogue at all. That is no less useful. As each states and restates their position and how it links into experience in the IGA, something is illuminated. The communications are open in many senses: open about what they experience and what their concerns are, open to the view of others, and open to response.

Separately, in a novel contribution, Anderson uses his imaginal response to group interaction in a film to illustrate a multiplicity of desires and disavowals of desires in a complex group interaction. There is a tradition of considering film in feminist studies and intersectionality. Anderson uses this to illuminate his understanding of clinical material in a way that shows a group analyst's thinking at work. He recognises the resonances in the fictional group around a common tension in a way that aligns with Haraway's work on diffraction, as I described in my chapter.

As described previously, the institutional setting may set constraints on the development of group-analytic training and theory. However, the institutional issues aside, as a corpus alone, Group Analysis, like Intersectionality, holds opposition to borders, including those between theoretical disciplines. This makes them ripe for learning from each other. Foulkes synthesised disciplines as different as Goldsteinian neurology, Gestalt psychology, classic psychoanalysis, anthropology, network theory, and Eliasian process sociology. Perhaps influenced by Elias in particular, he did not see a division between inside and outside (in some respects) in human development. Equally, as Nayak writes,

Intersectionality provides an argument for resistance to the split between theory and practice, centre and margin, individual and collective, subject and context, mind/body, and paternalistic service provider/professional and service recipient/user binary relations.

But what kind of resistance to splits? It is not quite right to say that Foulkes saw inside and outside as the same. That is a caricature. Group analysts recognise that patients come to them as individuals, albeit constituted in their relationships. In my chapter, I suggested that Barad went too far when they elided concepts that are by their nature different, while Haraway maintained a more sensible materialism. Inside and outside are not the same, although they are not as different as they may appear. Equally, simply saying there should be no borders between theories – and nothing can be internally coherent – cannot be right. The answer may come from Shelhi's suggestions. She says that she "seek[s] reconciliations that reflect the unity of diversity rather than the cohesion of undifferentiated clumped together parts". This is the difficult yet essential heart of the intersectional message, whether clinically or with theory. Group-analytic ideas have to be recognised as different from intersectional ideas in some regards and similar in others, each differing in a way that allows a dialogue between the ideas since they are not identical. It is through this process that they develop, and an intersectional group analysis can form.

Conclusion

In this edited collection, the authors show how they are re-orienting their group-analytic practice to consider intersectionality. They are doing this because of the suffering and repeat of exclusion and marginalisation, that comes from failing to do so. They do not suggest a theory that is deracinated from clinical work. That clinical work, whatever the setting, is informed by their thinking.

While there is much discussion of injustice, the authors have mentioned political concerns at times but only occasionally mention, in passing, justice. Justice may be a therapeutic, affective, reparative condition that seems quite far away from the expectations of the people coming for group-analytic psychotherapy – at least in its most complete experience. If it is something to be arrived at, some authors suggest a step-by-step approach, while others suggest an urgent need for something more radical.

The authors suggest, as new orienting concepts:

- Affectivism, as a way of tuning into moment-to-moment moves of shaming and negation and acting against them, in solidarity, to allow the value of oppressed voices to be heard – as an individual responsibility of each member of a group or training community.
- Recognising that bodies, which are not neutral sites but instead are socially-marked, are bearers of stress and traumatisation, and that they are a guide to what is going on.
- Valuing group polyphony as a method of avoiding pathologisation and allowing difference to be articulated constructively.
- Considering the group matrix as an intersectional matrix, with historical oppression woven into it, so that the dynamic matrix can be considered in full view and projective processes contained and understood rather than processes of rejection and marginalisation repeated.
- Making Group Analysis, theoretically, a slow-open group where new ideas can come in and be received with hospitality, and not just interacted with but intra-acted with, so that they are seen not as objects but living contributors, in so far as they have a clinical use.
- Recognising that racist social structures produce racist psychic structures, and a group-analytic training organisation in a racist society needs must consider its racist aspects.
- Insisting that changes to group-analytic theory, practice, and training cannot be at the level of slogans or buzzwords.

From Foulkes onwards, group analysts have recognised that individuals are social to their core. Now is the time for them to reaffirm this, with openness to new learning about how power operates in people's lives in highly personal ways. GROUP ANALYSIS CONTAINS THE POSSIBILITY OF BEING TRULY INTERSECTIONAL: WE HAVE TO RECOGNISE IT AND WORK HARD ON THAT BASIS.

References

Bacha, C. S. (2015) Commentary on Group Analytic Training and the Social Context: Who Is Influencing Whom? *Group Analysis*, 48(3): 368–378.

Campbell, K. (2004) The Promise of Feminist Reflexivities: Developing Donna Haraway's Project for Feminist Science Studies. *Hypatia*, 19(1): 162–182.

Crenshaw, K. (1989) Demarginalizing the Intersection of Race and Sex: A Black Feminist Critique of Antidiscrimination Doctrine, Feminist Theory, and Antiracist Politics. *The University of Chicago Legal Forum*, 140: 139–167.

Dalal, F. (1998) *Taking the Group Seriously: Towards a Post-Foulkesian Group Analytic Theory*. London: Jessica Kingsley.

Forrest, A. and Nayak, S. (2021) 'Should I Stay or Should I Go?' Group-Analytic Training: Inhabiting the Threshold of Ambivalence Is a Matter of Power, Privilege and Position. *Group Analysis*, 54(1): 55–68.

Hopper, E. (1996) The Social Unconscious in Clinical Work. *Group*, 20(1): 7–42.

Lorde, A. (2019 [1984]) *Sister Outsider*. London: Penguin Modern Classics.

Nayak, S. (2021) Black Feminist Intersectionality Is Vital to Group Analysis: Can Group Analysis Allow Outsider Ideas In? *Group Analysis*, 54(3): 337–353.

Nayak, S. (2022) An Intersectional Model of Reflection: Is Social Work Fit for Purpose in an Intersectionally Racist World? *Critical and Radical Social Work*, 10(2).

Spivak, G. C. (1988) Can the Subaltern Speak? In Nelson, C. and Grossberg, L. (eds.) *Marxism and the Interpretation of Culture*. Basingstoke: Macmillan Education, pp. 271–313.

Index

Note: Page numbers in **bold** refer to tables.

For Product Safety Concerns and Information please contact our EU
representative GPSR@taylorandfrancis.com
Taylor & Francis Verlag GmbH, Kaufingerstraße 24, 80331 München, Germany

www.ingramcontent.com/pod-product-compliance
Lightning Source LLC
Chambersburg PA
CBHW060309220326
41598CB00027B/4285